JimsHealthAndMu

The 6-Week Resistance Training Book

Lose weight & tone muscle efficiently with this exercise challenge & simple diet advice. A method that will always work.

James Atkinson

CONTENTS

Section 1

Is this workout book for you?

Most people who join a gym, buy a set of resistance bands or a weight set have the goal of muscle toning and fat loss in mind. This is an excellent start, as lowering body fat and increasing muscle tone will set an unshakable foundation for the development of all aspects of fitness. This book is for anyone who has ever wanted to make positive, meaningful visual and functional changes to their fitness levels.

There are several aspects of fitness, including cardio health, flexibility, strength, endurance and body composition. Most types of exercise target progression in one of these components more than the others. This guide has a focus on body composition and strength, but also considers cardio health and endurance along the way, using resistance training and diet as its main tool kit.

Six weeks is not a long time in the health and fitness game, but we can make excellent progress with fat loss and muscle tone in this timeframe with a few simple actions. But simple doesn't mean easy!

If you want to lose body fat and tone muscle to attain a healthy physique visually and functionally, it will challenge you in mind and body.

We geared this workout book to help you:

- Reduce body fat percentage
- Increase muscle tone
- Become stronger
- Become healthier
- Stay consistent and disciplined for the long term

The last point on the list above is by far the most important skill to develop, as the other points are a by-product of this one.

If you see it through, you will be rewarded, not only with the new physique you have earned, but with the knowledge and experience you have gained along the way. This experience can have a truly profound and positive effect in all aspects of your life.

This guide can serve as a gateway to success in improved physical health and indeed mental health too.

It's not all about body image, it's about health, function, balance and longevity. We are all dealt a hand when we are born and it's up to us how we choose to play it. I always assume that everyone would like to be the best version of themselves in body and mind, meaning a development of mental robustness and physical capability. The only barrier to this is not having a direction or, indeed, the knowledge to do so. If you do not agree with me on this, the book is probably not for you, as you may disagree with the overall message and practices inside. If you are with me, I'm excited to have you along and truly look forward to hearing of your success!

Despite our differences, we are all made of the same stuff. We all have the ability to make choices. We all have muscle and fat, and we all have to eat to survive. If we eat the right food and challenge our bodies in the right way, we can attain our potential in health and fitness.

There are no shortcuts to body composition change, and the road is almost never linear, but believe it or not, the journey starts as soon as the thought that we want to change crosses our minds.

This is a no-nonsense guide on how to change body composition, meaning, reduce body fat and tone muscle using diet and resistance exercise.

These days, it seems there are a multitude of approaches to getting this done, some easier than others, but the truth is that the age old approach of correct diet and exercise, practiced consistently, is the most effective and sustainable way. As long as the human body continues to work the way it does, this will always be the case.

If you are still with me, let's get started! Today is the day, so carpe diem!

Introduction

It's easy to become confused and overwhelmed with the many conflicting ideas about fat loss and muscle toning. This doesn't just apply to the beginner in the fitness game; it also applies to the veterans.

Variations in training and diet advice are ubiquitous and diverse. Add to this the obscene market value of the fitness industry, the reach and influence of social media, and you have the perfect storm of people cashing in on the next "ground breaking health hack" to further add to the confusion.

I can see the irony! You could argue that I am part of the problem by publishing a fitness book with a title such as this one, but here's my justification.

My name is James Atkinson (Jim to my readers and friends). I've been into fitness and exercise for most of my life and my experience has an extreme range, from skinny to competing bodybuilder, from overweight to endurance runner, I have formal qualifications in advanced fitness instruction, and I'm an Amazon bestselling author in the fitness niche.

Before taking advice from a potential mentor, it's important to know their background. I've faced common challenges in this game and want to share my experience with you, not brag about my accomplishments. At this point, I want to thank you for your purchase and let you know I am always willing to help where I can with your fitness journey. I've met some great people this way and followed their progress over ten years in some cases. Replying to emails from people like you is one highlight of this job.

I'm a real person who has experienced the ups and downs of fitness; I am not a ghost-writer, and I don't use a pseudonym. I'm passionate about my subject and write from personal experience. I've had great success with fitness, but part of the journey to great success was often great failure and I have that too. If I can share relevant, personal experiences of my failures to help you avoid potential problems, then this is no failure!

I've experimented with different types of training, diets, and theories, like many others, but I've learned that the basics are the key to achieving sustainable, meaningful fitness results. Master the basics and you will see through all the hype and marketing techniques that are likely to throw you off your path.

Let's talk "body transformation" and the basics. For the purpose of this fitness book, body transformation is to mean changing the state of the body by changing its composition. We will consider two variables. These being body fat and muscle mass.

Body fat

Body fat is usually measured as a percentage. We can calculate this in several ways, including:

- BMI
- Smart scales
- Callipers
- DEXA
- Hydrostatic weighing

But, we want basic and simple! The body fat that we are concerned about when looking to change the condition and shape of our body is that which covers us all over. Some people have more body fat around the abdomen, some have more around the hips and some have more around the lower back. We are all different. The one thing that unites us, however, is that we all have a covering of body fat. Some have more than others. The more we have, the less visible our muscles are and the more at risk of serious illness and health issues we are. By increasing muscle strength and tone whilst also reducing body fat percentage, we will see and feel relatively quick results. Skeletal muscle becomes more pronounced and as body fat decreases, these muscles also become more visible.

Muscle mass

Muscle mass is the amount of muscle we have on our bodies. This covers all muscle types, such as skeletal muscle, deep muscle, and cardiac muscle. There are some muscle types that we can't train, but the ones that we can, we will focus on; these being skeletal muscle and cardiac muscle.

The connection between body fat and muscle mass

There is a connection between the increase of muscle and increased speed of fat loss. The most basic way to explain this is: The biggest amount of energy output per day for most people is from their basal metabolic rate. Basal Metabolic rate or "BMR" is energy or "calories" burned through the body's basic functions, like breathing and metabolising food.

If we have more lean muscle mass, it takes more energy for our bodies to function. This means we burn more calories with more muscle. For this reason, this guide focuses heavily on resistance training.

Diet

Misunderstanding of diet is common. We are all "on a diet" at every point in our lives. Simply put, our diet is what we eat. If we educate ourselves in choosing and eating food that has useful nutrition and is low in non-useful nutrition in the right quantities, we can expect to lower body fat percentages to healthy levels. If we live by this, we will never need to "go on a fat loss diet" ever again. This is sustainability.

If we add the right type of exercise, we can expect to see an increase in muscle tone, muscle strength, and better function.

Why 6 weeks?

Some people will see results within as little as a week, but a week is not long enough to see a meaningful change with fat loss and muscle growth. The effects of consistency are exponential to a point that extends over several months or even years. It's been said many times before that a habit is established if an action is consistently taken over a 4-week period. Here, diet and exercise are the habits.

If we do everything right and stay consistent with our diet and training, we will see excellent results after 4 weeks, but another 2 weeks on top of this is likely to see much more noticeable results when it comes to our body composition. Although the routine in this guide is set for six weeks, it can be sustained indefinitely to maintain or continue development. There may be a point where progress slows down or stops. If you get to this point, you will need to tweak the training or diet slightly. I'm here to help with this, so give me a shout if you need someone to bounce ideas off. It's worth mentioning that if you get to a plateau such as this, you are doing an outstanding job.

The idea of the first six weeks it to establish routine, healthy habits and achieve physical and visual changes to our bodies. With these achievements, we can take the information in this guide and continue with our progress.

More information and fitness tips

There is enough information in this fitness book to absorb and implement, but I want you to get results and I'm here to help you get to where you want to be in fitness! If you are not where you want to be and can't see a path, I have a free podcast where I chat about common issues and give advice on how to overcome and progress. I'd love to squeeze all the advice for everyone into a single guide, but this can detract from a goal and causing overwhelm. I've seen it many times and been there myself. Too many ideas can cause paralysis, causing no action to be taken at all.

If podcasts are your thing, I have one that addresses common issues with fitness progression. Each episode is read by myself highlighting a specific topic, giving actionable advice based on experience. Episode length is around twenty minutes. So let's chat! Get a coffee on, drop by and have a listen at:

AudioFitTest.com

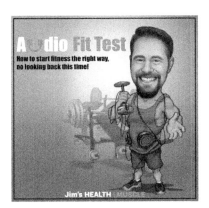

Health Check

Before you embark on any fitness routine, please consult your doctor or physiotherapist. If you have any health conditions, always check if the type of exercise and exercise choices you intend to involve yourself with.

1.   Do not exercise if you are unwell.

2.   Stop if you feel pain, and if the pain does not subside, consult your doctor or physiotherapist.

3.   Do not exercise if you have taken alcohol or had a large meal in the last few hours.

4.   If you are taking medication, please check with your doctor to make sure it is okay for you to exercise.

5.   If in doubt at all, please check with your doctor or physiotherapist first – you may even want to take this routine and go through it with them. It may be helpful to ask for a blood pressure, cholesterol and weight check. You can then have these taken again in a few months to see the benefit.

Body weight or body fat?

For many people, the concept of weighing themselves on a set of scales is fundamental to a body transformation or general fitness goal. When someone tells me they have lost X amount of weight, I first congratulate them, then I always ask for more information.

The information that their "weight loss" achievement gives me is that I know they are dedicated to their goal and are more than capable of achieving their potential with fitness.

If, on the other hand, someone tells me they reduced their body fat by 10 per cent, it gives me a bit more information. It first tells me that their mind-set is different, that they are dedicated to their goal and are more than capable of achieving their potential with fitness. But it also tells me that they are focused on body composition change rather than body weight, which means they have an interest in maintaining, growing or toning muscle to give them extra health and fitness benefits.

Why is this important?

When someone says they want to "lose weight", they really mean they want to "lose body fat". Reducing body weight and reducing body fat are two different things.

To lose body weight, we can cut our hair, nails, go to the toilet or even remove a limb, so the scales are the perfect measurement device for this result. This ticks the box for a weight loss goal.

Skeletal muscle like our biceps, quads, glutes and lats are also part of our body weight. If we train these with resistance exercise, they will become denser. This means they will be heavier, which gives us more body weight. But having these muscles gives us a better opportunity to get rid of unwanted body fat.

It is possible for someone to stay the same weight and be in a lot better shape, visually and internally. Eating the correct food at the right amounts is a great start, but if we don't challenge the muscles of our body at the same time, we could be a lot lighter and still be unfit and out of shape.

I fully understand that some may think that "being in shape" is superficial, but being in shape offers far more than a mere visual effect. There are an amazing amount of health benefits that walk hand in hand with it. At the start of a fitness venture, if you were offered the chance to look good naked or to just get to a certain body fat percentage, regardless of the visual and health benefits, what would you choose?

Someone at 15 percent body fat who has a base of muscle tone all over will not only look in better shape than someone at 15% body fat who has not been training with resistance, they will be stronger and fitter too, they will also have an easier time with further progression as they have more muscle mass to boost energy expenditure with their BMR (basal metabolic rate). More on BMR later.

In my experience, the term "building muscle" tends to put some people off this whole idea, as looking like a bodybuilder is not what they want. But until someone actually tries to look like a bodybuilder through diet and training, it's not really appreciated how hard it is to get this result. Attaining a bodybuilder physique doesn't happen by accident. If this is one of your reservations, let me put your mind at rest; the training and diet advice in this guide is not geared towards bodybuilders. It is geared towards fat burning, developing lean muscle tone and function.

There are differing opinions on the ideal body fat percentage range, and whether we like it or not, gender is a variable which widens these parameters. A male trainer will find it easier to build muscle and reduce body fat percentage than a female, as the male has a more suited hormonal tool kit for the job.

From a medical point of view, a healthy body fat percentage for a male is around 20 – 25 percent and for a female, it is around 30 – 35 percent. At the higher ends of these suggestions, (25 and 35 percent) we would see little muscle definition, if any.

Regardless of gender, the food we eat is metabolised in the same way, so food choices do not need to differ for a body composition change

Both male and female trainers can achieve an impressive, lean, strong physique, and where body fat percentage is concerned, this starts at around the 20 percent mark. The training and diet advice in this guide will help you to achieve this. Lowering body fat below 20 percent may need a more measured approach on the diet side of things. For some perspective, body fat below 20 percent on a toned physique is the type of composition you would expect to see on a hype fuelled fitness publication.

The basic principal

I want to keep this guide simple but effective. Sure, there are scientific explanations and deep dives into exact macronutrients required, training variations that target specific function in different muscle groups and optimal training conditions. But we are not dieticians, human biologists, or Olympic athletes; we simply want to burn fat and tone muscle to give us a body composition change or "transformation" and reap the many health benefits that come with it.

So how do we go about this with minimal fuss?

The basic principle

"Calories in, calories out" is a phrase we have probably all heard for weight loss goals. Meaning we have to eat fewer calories than we burn to lose weight. This is true and always will be. However, there is a better way of looking at it, which is:

"Supporting fuel goes in and we aim for more energy expended,"

We should eat to "support" our fitness goals. As we will train for muscle growth and toning, we will need to support this with quality food. There are two parts of the puzzle, and the first is diet and nutrition. Don't worry, this is easier than you think by following a few basic rules. The other part is exercise. Again, there are a few things to consider, but the simple steps in the planning phase will take you through this.

The basic principles to change your body composition are to eat quality food, exercise regularly for muscle growth, and be consistent. The hardest part is staying consistent, but with correct planning, it makes this a whole lot easier, hence the upcoming highlights of planning.

More energy expended

Resistance training is ideal for muscle growth and tone, and if performed regularly and with the right intensity, it can burn more calories than cardio training sessions of the same length. During a resistance training session, the calories burned are generally less than a cardio session, but studies have shown that calories burned post resistance workout are greater than that of cardio sessions, so, technically, the training session continues long after we put our resistance equipment away.

Like cardio exercise, not all resistance exercises are made equal. For the purpose of this book, we want to get the most out of our resistance training sessions to burn more calories in each resistance session, this is why we will focus mainly on compound exercises. These are exercises that require more than one muscle group to perform a single rep. Using compound exercises gives us more intensity in our workouts, more energy expended per rep and a better opportunity to work with each major muscle group in a single or split session.

Compound exercises can be performed with all types of resistance, including bodyweight, exercise bands, barbells, and dumbbells.

What about cardio training?

Cardio training is anything that exercises the heart and lungs over a sustained period of time, walking, jogging, running, rowing, cycling, etc. The best way to look at cardio exercise is not that it burns fat, but it expends energy. The longer we spend performing a cardio activity, the more energy we use. If we couple this with a caloric deficit, over time, we will lose body fat.

Cardio training has many benefits, one of which is to develop the capability of the heart and lungs. We can all benefit from this. Sessions of steady state cardio and interval training are also great for burning energy. But this type of training is best used as a secondary or supplementary exercise method alongside resistance training if the training goal is for fat loss and all over muscle development.

The issue with focusing on cardio exercise exclusively is that it neglects to target many major muscle groups. Focusing exclusively on cardio exercise neglects to challenge many major muscle groups, resulting in minimal development and often diminished function.

With this said, cardio training is an excellent addition to any resistance workout routine to increase the calorie deficit further.

What to eat

It's far more efficient to control the calories, or energy we put into our bodies than trying to expend the calories that we have taken on, in order to lose body fat.

"I'll eat this chocolate bar. It's ok, I'll just do a bit more in the gym or go for a run to burn it off."

Anyone who exercises regularly has said, or at least had thoughts similar to this at some point. Based on a 300 calorie chocolate bar, with this mind-set, you would have to add an extra thirty minutes, averagely paced jog to your existing workout session to be close to offsetting the extra calorie intake.

Before we begin this section, I believe it's important to understand that burning off "bad calories" is not as easy as we think. These extra thirty minute jogs can really add up, and we should all remember this when we have the opportunity to indulge in treats.

Eating correctly is essential for anybody composition change. There are "industry standard", age-old methods for estimating calories and macro nutrients to guarantee results with fat loss and muscle development, which are highlighted at the end of this section. But from my experience, most people look at this and decide they don't have the time or they feel it is too complicated to implement.

This is a fair point. Following this calculation and figuring out the weight of food, macros and meal timings is a lot of ongoing work. It is, however, worthwhile to persevere with the process, as it's the very best way to get to where we want to be in the quickest time. But it is still a big commitment.

Over the years I've been helping people with diet and exercise, I've come to understand that trainers wishing to achieve fat loss and muscle tone through exercise would rather focus on the exercise routines rather than the diet. But correct diet is the deciding factor in body shape and body composition.

I've been approached many times by trainers that ask for further advice using words to the effect of:

"I'm much stronger now, but I've still got this belly"

Or

"I've been training so hard for a while now and I'm still carrying this extra fat. This training doesn't work"

The answer is always:

"What's your diet like?"

Explaining the whole calculation of where to start to get a solid estimate of macro nutrients each day, not only makes me feel like a total bore, but I can honestly say that I've never come across anyone who didn't; at worst state that they were not going to do that and at best pretend to be interested as a matter of curtesy. These days there are many online diet calculators out there that simplify the process, but even making the most of the data from these apps can be tiresome.

I'm confident that ninety-nine percent of people don't want to use calculations and weigh food at every mealtime, so I've come up with a few simple rules to follow to make the nutrition part of this plan easier.

- Eat quality, low processed food
- Nutritional ratios
- Practice portion control

Quality nutrition

"Eat less and train more" or "fewer calories in and more calories out" is a great starting mind-set, but it goes a bit deeper than this if fat loss and muscle development is the goal. The calories that we put in should be high quality, low processed foods. There are several reasons for this. The first is that there are fewer ingredients making up good quality whole foods. We often find hidden empty calories, like flavourings and preservatives in processed convenience foods. You know what you are getting with a chicken breast when compared to a chicken nugget, for example.

The next is that there are more nutrients in whole foods like brown rice, granary bread for example. If we compare brown rice to white rice, the brown rice has the bran left on it, as it has not been milled. White rice has been processed to remove this fibre.

Why is this important? As the brown rice has more to it, it takes more energy for the body to process, so this means we would not only feel fuller for longer eating brown rice than we would eating white rice, but we would also be burning more calories in the digestion process. If we are eating whole foods like this all the time, this really does add up and helps tremendously towards our fitness goals!

If we are eating high quality, low processed foods, there are many of these that we have to eat significantly more of to reach the same amount of calories as high-calorie, processed foods. For example, if you ate 150g of chicken breast (which is around the size of an average chicken breast) you would consume about 250 calories. If you ate 150g of cheese pizza (which is about a slice) you would be consuming around 400 calories.

As you can see, the difference is significant. It's also worth considering that when having chicken breast with a meal, most people would only have one, but who has a single slice of pizza in a single sitting?

Chicken breast, a whole food, contains nutrients like protein and calories that our bodies can use to build muscle and burn fat. The calories in the average pizza slice are made up of processed foods like pizza dough, which is technically white bread, a processed food with very little to offer in support of our fitness goal. Cheese is not a "bad" food, but it has many variants and is generally high in calories to weight ratio.

Nutritional ratios

Selecting only quality foods that help fuel our bodies is the first step, but we also know that we need to be at a calorie deficit to help us lose body fat. But not all quality, whole foods are equal when it comes to volume vs calorie content. For example, nuts and some types of cheese are whole foods, but they are also very calorie dense, so these types of foods need to be eaten in moderation.

For the purpose of this fitness goal, as we are training with resistance and we aim to feed our muscles, we need to also eat quality protein and carbohydrates.

Carbohydrates should make up fifty percent of each meal, protein should make up twenty-five percent and vegetables rich in vitamins and minerals should make up the other twenty-five percent.

So, in theory, this is what the ratios should look like on a plate at each meal:

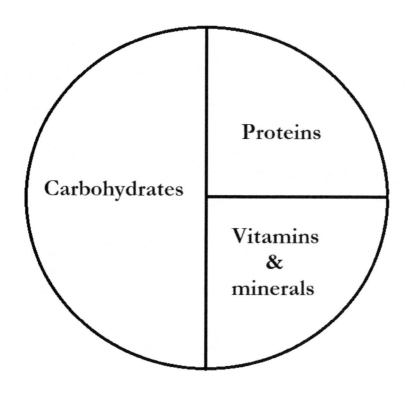

This may sound controversial, as there is no mention of fat. Fat is actually an essential nutrition that our bodies need. Omitting fat sources from our main meals has a few benefits in relation to our goals, however.

- Fat has double the amount of calories as protein and carbohydrates per gram
- Essential fats can be found in meats, fish, and dairy
- High-quality fats can be found in snack options
- Omitting fat from our meals will dramatically help with the goal of eating at a calorie deficit.

The ratio theory of 50 percent carbs, 25 percent protein and 25 percent vitamins and minerals per meal holds up if we are training with resistance exercise regularly as we have the carbohydrates for energy, protein for muscle building and vitamins and minerals to help with function.

It may also seem shocking that carbohydrates dominate the ratios. Carbohydrates are somewhat demonised in this day and age. They get the blame for excessive fat gain and are often cut out of diets as the first port of call when trying to lose weight. But carbohydrates are misunderstood. Good quality, whole grain carbohydrates, eaten in the right quantities, are your friends for bodyweight composition changes involving resistance training. It is only when we aim to drop body fat to below twenty to fifteen per cent that we may need to look at cutting whole food carbohydrate ratios.

Portion control

Eating smaller volumes of any food will reduce calories going in. But if we take the above point of "quality nutrition" and practice this at every mealtime, some trainers are likely to cover the portion control aspect of diet by default.

I've observed that people's views on portion control can vary significantly from one individual to another, and it's been an interest of mine for quite some time. There is always the option of following the calculations and working out your individual estimate of daily calories and macronutrients needed for weight loss, then using the scales to weigh every meal.

This is the most accurate way to start eating correct portion sizes, but it's a time-consuming process. I always recommend this to anyone as it gives us much valuable information. But for those who want to minimise fuss, there is another way.

- A deck of playing cards
- A small box of matches
- A tablespoon
- The palm of your hand

Are the tools that you need to play this game.

For each meal, and using the ratios mentioned in the "Nutritional ratios" point, you can use these tools to determine portion sizes per meal:

Carbohydrates – Should fit in the palm of your hand. A slice of wholegrain/granary bread is a good example of this measure.

Protein – Should be the size of a standard deck of playing cards. A small chicken breast or a portion of mackerel fillets are good examples of this.

High calorie, high value whole foods – Should be the size of a small matchbox. A slice of cheese or a portion of nuts are good examples of this.

Vitamins and minerals – Leafy greens and dark green vegetables are high in nutritional value and very low in calories. This means that you do not need to worry too much about your portion sizes here, so add these to your meals in order to bulk them out and add variation, within reason.

Table spoons – When food is hard to measure against a deck of cards, a box of matches or the palm of your hand, tablespoons are useful. We can use heaped table spoons to get similar portion sizes.

- Four heaped table spoons – Carbohydrates such as rice, pasta, mashed potatoes/ sweet potatoes, etc.
- Two heaped tablespoons – Proteins such as minced, lean meats, lentils, beans, cottage cheese.
- One heaped table spoon – High value, high-calorie foods used for snacks such as nuts, grated cheese, avocado and dried fruit. We can count quality oils used for cooking and dressings such as extra virgin olive oil on this portion size measurement, too.

Ninety-nine percent of the time, using this method of measuring foods will work well and if we are strict with the food choices we make (we choose quality nutrition), going over these portion size suggestions will not be too much of a problem.

Meal and snack frequency

Eating 3 meals per day with 2 snacks between meals (one snack between breakfast and lunch and one between lunch and evening meal) is ideal for the goal of this book. Here's the theory; eating regularly will keep hunger levels low, regulate insulin levels and reduce, or even put a stop to over eating convenience food with low nutritional value.

Breakfast, lunch and evening meal should be standard, but if we are following this guide, we will be spending more energy than usual due to the workouts. Our bodies will need the energy we are putting in to repair and recover, and we'll probably be consuming fewer calories than usual. This is where snacking between meals is useful. This eating schedule is one of the most difficult parts for a lot of people as most of us have regular day jobs and lead busy lives. But finding the time to eat at this cadence should be something we all aim for. We need this fuel, so we should do our very best to make it happen.

Meal and snack variation

Planning meals and variation is a time-consuming process, especially if you are new to doing so. If, however, you have a balanced nutritional plan to support your training goals for a single day, you can repeat every single day. This will make the entire process easier. Athletes and trainers who compete in sporting events often use this approach. By not having to workout macro nutrients and energy intake from every meal, every day, these trainers can stick to a single daily meal plan in the knowledge that they will not have to revisit calculations for the next few weeks leaving them extra headspace and time to focus on their training.

Meal plan example

Here is a daily meal plan example that contains around 2130 calories. This can be used as it is or it can be tweaked to suit your personal needs. A lot of people will think this is a lot of food and is more than they would normally eat. The volume may be higher than many are used to, but the energy contained in the full plan may be lower. All the food listed is high in nutritional value.

If you decide to give this a go, but find that it is too much, simply cut out the snacks or reduce the portion sizes. If you are training regularly and with the correct intensity, you may find you are hungry between meals, this is the reason for the snack options.

Hydration

Water is the transport for the nutrition we put into our bodies, so its role in body composition change is vital. We should all drink water throughout the day and get into the habit of taking it with us as part of our nutrition plan. For the purpose of this guide and fitness results intended, I will state that energy drinks are not useful for us at all. Water is by far our best choice.

Breakfast

- 250g Greek yoghurt – 400 calories
- 60g rolled oats – 230 calories
- 50g blueberries – 30 calories

This is an inexpensive, convenient and well balanced nutritious breakfast. Greek yoghurt can be bought in pots around the 500g mark. This means a full pot is breakfast for two days. Supermarkets branded rolled oats are cheap and will last a few weeks. Any fresh fruit can be used to make this breakfast more interesting, but blueberries are a great example.

A bonus tip – Mix the oats, yoghurt and blueberries together in a bowl on day one. Day two, use the yoghurt pot with the left over yoghurt from day one to mix in the oats and fruit. Do yourself a favour and save on washing up dishes!

Snack

- 30g Almonds – 165 calories

30 grams of almonds are about 20 nuts. You don't have to count these out every time, but it's good to get a gauge on the amount by counting them out once. Check what 20 almonds look like in your hand and remember this or find a small pot that fits 20 almonds inside and use this as a measure going forward.

Lunch

- 150g Can of tuna – 170 calories
- 125g brown rice (cooked weight) – 100 calories
- 1 tbsp. of mayonnaise – 90 calories
- Ground black pepper – NA
- Leafy green salad – NA

Natural herbs and spices do not really need to be moderated as they are so low in calories and the amount we use is negligible, so we can experiment in this area to make the food we eat more interesting.

Leafy green salad also does not need to be moderated, as the nutritional value that comes from this far outweighs the few calories it offers.

You can make a vegetarian replacement for tuna by mashing up cooked chickpeas, mixing a few herbs or spices in, and adding the mayo. Even for non-vegetarian eaters, this is a good option.

Snack

- 1 Slice of granary bread – 120 calories
- 1 tbsp. Natural peanut butter – 100 calories

Toasting the bread before spreading the peanut butter makes this a whole lot more interesting.

Dinner

- 200g Chicken breast – 330 calories
- 250g Large jacket potato – 240 calories
- 100g Stir-fried broccoli in 1tbsp vegetable oil - 155 calories

Bonus tip – Marinade the chicken in garlic, chilli and lime juice before cooking. Flame grilled, this is very tasty! Any seasoning can be used on the chicken, but it's best to use seasoning that is natural. Many ready-made packet seasonings have lots of preservatives, sugars and salt. This is something to be aware of.

Broccoli can be switched for any green vegetables such as asparagus, runner beans or mangetout. Stir-frying is quick and easy, but makes these greens pop with flavour. You can also slice up some spring onion and throw this into the pan for even more flavour.

A vegetarian replacement for chicken breast could be a homemade bean and quinoa burger. There are good ready-made vegetarian options out there, but if we create our own meals from raw ingredients, we know exactly what's going in to the end product and it will be far cheaper.

A skill to learn and some perspective

Making healthy food choices starts with educating ourselves on what's "good", how to identify nutritional value and a balance of macronutrients. This is an ongoing process for everyone, but the more we practise it, the easier it will become.

Choosing the correct nutrition is one thing, but learning to cook and prepare food is an invaluable asset to our fitness goals. Once we choose the right balance and portion sizes of nutrition, we can look at different ways to cook, season and serve this to make some really interesting meals.

To finish this section, I would like to use the above daily diet plan example to reinforce the point of portion control being fulfilled by default and to also highlight that "calories in vs calories out" has more to it than that.

Here is some perspective: This daily diet plan example contains around 2300 calories of nutrition that will support our fitness goal of fat loss and muscle tone. I can tell you that a single 13.5" pepperoni pizza from a globally popular pizzeria holds around 2642 calories that will not support our fitness goals of fat loss and muscle tone.

For those who want to take it to the next level

As advertised, here are the calculations for those who want to take it to the next level. I appreciate that this is not for everyone and that it goes against the "keep it simple" nature of this particular guide, but I feel it should be added as it is the most accurate way to start a nutritional plan for your specific situation.

If you follow the advice in this guide and you get results, but after a while you plateau, you may want to take a look at this and reassess your diet.

Here's some algebra!

BMR

This is our "basal metabolic rate". It's the estimated measure of energy burned when we are at rest. We need to work this out first:

Male: (Height in CM X 6.25) + (weight in KG X 9.99) – (age X 4.92) +5

Female: (Height in CM X 6.25) + (weight in KG X 9.99) – (age X 4.92) – 161

Activity level

Some people are more active than others and this has an effect on calories burned, so we have to consider it. Once we have our BMR, we can use it for the next step. Activity levels and the BMR result are used in the next calculation:

Little to no exercise: BMR X 1.2

Light exercise (1-3 days per week): BMR X 1.375

Moderate exercise (3-5 days per week): BMR X 1.55

Heavy exercise (6 – 7 days per week): BMR X 1.725

This figure will give us the estimated amount of supporting calories we need to maintain our current composition. To lose weight, we would need to eat fewer calories than this number.

This equation with me as an example:

I've rounded any fractions in the equation to the nearest full number. This is something that you should also do.

Gender - Male

Height – 180 cm

Weight – 90 kg

Age – 42

BMR = (180 X 6.25 = 1125) + (90 X 9.99 = 899) – (42 X 4.29 = 180) +5 = 1850

BMR: 1850

Moderate exercise: 1850 X 1.5 = 2775

I need **2775** calories of quality nutrition to maintain.

So, if I wanted to lose weight, I would need to eat less than this. The example diet plan in this section is ideal.

If we follow the rest of the nutritional advice in this book, stick to high value, low processed foods, and follow the exercise routines, as you will see, it's easier to eat at a calorie deficit than you might think.

With this said. Diet and calorie intake are different for everyone; this calculation is a "best guess" approach that we can work from. If you are finding fat loss to be slow going (less than 3lbs per week), you can reduce your estimate by 10 percent, try it for a week and then reassess. Maybe you need to add a daily cardio session to up calorie expenditure rather than cut out more food if you are struggling with hunger. There are a few things that you can do, but this is a great starting point.

Workout methods

There are lots of ways to train with resistance. Because this guide is focused on body composition change, full body workouts and split training, using compound exercises are going to be highlighted as the best option. For clarity:

Full body workouts

Full body workouts are workouts with exercises that challenge every major muscle group in the body during a single or split session. This could be a traditional "sets and reps" or a "circuit training" approach.

Split training

Split training is a workout method that includes exercises to challenge every major muscle group in the body split over several sessions per week. In this guide a split training session will have two parts. Each part is performed on alternate days. This is known as a "2 day split".

Exercise method

Compound exercises are exercises that target multiple muscle groups during a single rep. These exercises are widely considered to be the best choices for strength and muscle gains and in the interest of energy expenditure (fat loss), they are generally far superior to isolation exercises.

In this guide the options will be:

- Full body workouts using sets and reps
- Full body workouts using circuit training
- Split routines utilising the above options

The type of resistance training you want to do depends on a few things. The first and most fundamental is the accessibility of the exercise equipment. If you have access to a public gym, then you will have access to most, if not all of the equipment needed to explore any of the options in this book. The same is true if you have your own home gym.

The most lightweight, space saving and affordable option is bodyweight training or resistance band training. These types of training options can be done from home too.

Bodyweight

It is possible to perform compound exercises for all major muscle groups in the body using bodyweight and gravity. Most exercise using bodyweight require no equipment, but there are some muscle groups that need a platform to work from. For example, the back muscles (latissimus dorsi) are a muscle group that need either a rowing movement or a pull down movement to engage as part of a compound exercise. This means we need a solid bar raised off the floor that can take our weight.

Resistance band workouts

Resistance bands are extremely versatile and can be used for all the compound exercises mentioned in this guide. As mentioned, they are easily stored and pretty affordable. Resistance bands can be for all types of training, so they are a great bit of kit to have.

Barbell workouts

Barbells range in size and weight. The size of these things can be inconvenient if they are being used for home workouts. They are also plate loaded, so extra space is needed for the storage of these. A barbell however is the resistance equipment of choice for many strength trainers, bodybuilders and veteran trainers everywhere as they can be used with great effect for compound exercises.

Dumbbell workouts

Dumbbells are, again, bulky and take up a lot of space, but they are great for compound exercises. The difference between barbells and dumbbells is that they are independent, so dumbbells also strengthen stabiliser muscles. They also give the option of using a slightly wider range of movement on exercises as hands are not set in a single position through a lift.

Multi workouts

Multi workouts are exercise sessions that use any variation of resistance training. We could use a bodyweight exercise for chest, a resistance band exercise for back, a barbell exercise for shoulders etc.

There are several reasons for opting to use multi workouts. The most obvious is availability of workout equipment. Barbells are not practical for everyone, especially if you are planning to workout from home.

Certain exercise movements with certain equipment might not be suitable for some trainers. For example bodyweight training is the most accessible for everyone as it requires very little training equipment, but bodyweight exercise can be very challenging and exercises such as push ups or bodyweight row may not be achievable, so these can be substituted with resistance band chest press and resistance band row respectively to target the same muscle groups.

On the other side of the same coin, trainers may outgrow bodyweight exercises and no longer find them challenging enough. These trainers may wish to increase the workload on muscle groups by adding more resistance to a chest press with tougher resistance bands, or, if the equipment is available, use a loaded barbell to their chest press exercise.

Workload & intensity

Workload and training intensity is often an aspect of fitness progression that trainers get wrong which interferes with results. As we are all different, it can take some trial and error and some time, not only to find the correct intensity for us, but to understand how our bodies respond to training.

There are several components that make up workload and intensity:

- Frequency of exercise
- Volume of exercise
- Intensity
- Time of training session

Frequency of exercise

Frequency of workout is defined by how often we perform exercise sessions. Regular resistance exercise will promote consistent energy expenditure over time. Training every day would be great, but this may be a bit much for some people, depending on their current fitness level. Training three times per week is probably the minimum we should aim for.

It is possible to exercise twice per day for some trainers. If this is within your means and you'd like to explore the possibilities, I would suggest that a resistance training session is performed in the morning and a cardio session such as a brisk walk is performed later in the day.

Volume of exercise

Volume is defined by how many sets and reps are performed per session, along with the resistance level within the sets and reps range. Volume is broken down further into the volume on every exercise. A good starting point is three sets per exercise and five to seven exercises per session.

The resistance level is defined by how much resistance is used per repetition (rep). This is very subjective as everyone will be at differing levels of fitness. Resistance level, or weight you lift per rep can be tracked fairly easily, but to identify an effective resistance, we need to look at intensity.

Intensity

Intensity is linked to volume in that there will be an effective range of resistance that we should work inside. If the volume of exercise is sound, but the intensity is too low, we will not achieve optimal results as we did not challenge our muscles enough during the workout. If the volume is sound and the intensity is too high, we may struggle to complete a workout.

The correct intensity means we are sufficiently challenged throughout the exercise session. During the last few reps of each set, we should be at about sixty to seventy per cent of exhaustion. Exhaustion meaning that we fail to perform another rep with good exercise form. For newer trainers, this may take some trial and error during the early stages of this training routine.

Working out with correct intensity is a common mistake. Our muscle groups need to be challenged enough each workout. If we exercise with correct form and are on the edge of losing this form near the end of our set, this is the correct intensity. If we get this right, our resistance level becomes somewhat irrelevant. For example, if I can perform a barbell bench press with a 10kg bar for 12 reps but struggle to maintain good exercise form on the last few reps and you can do the same but with a barbell weighing 100kg, we are both working with the right intensity.

Time of training session

The time it takes to complete a workout. This is less important for the purpose of this guide, but it is still a useful measurement, especially with circuit training as heart rate will be elevated for longer per session. Each training session when using single exercises in a "sets and reps" format should last between forty-five minutes to an hour. Circuit training sessions can generally last as little as thirty minutes as the intensity is greater due to the prolonged sets value. But as long as we are completing our planned workload, the time it takes should not be a major concern at this point.

What's the plan?

Exercise and diet are the key ingredients for long-term health and fitness progress, but planning is extremely important in order to make this happen. Before you decide to make a single meal set out by the guidelines in this book, or indeed perform a single rep of an exercise, you should plan for at least one week ahead.

It's not the single healthy meal or the single exercise session that will change anything, it's the compounded effect of many meals and exercise sessions over time that makes the difference. When you are ready, you can follow these steps.

There are three steps to this process:

Step one – Identifying the right foods and plan your meals

Identifying the correct food may be an ongoing process for some, so stick to the basics at the beginning. Decide what you will eat for breakfast, lunch, evening meal and snacks. Go shopping and make sure you have enough of this food in your cupboards to last you at least a week.

Although variety of food does help, you do not have to change the meals you eat from day to day, provided you have the right quantity and nutrition ratios each day you can work from the same menu on a daily basis. It's often easier to stay organised and remain consistent this way as it takes up less headspace.

The last thing to be said about diet is that this word should be associated with your lifestyle and it's not a temporary thing. The correct diet for our fitness goal is one that is nutritionally balanced, calorie controlled and sustainable for the long term. When good diet and exercise habits are firmly established and we are happy with our fitness results, we can maybe think about working in a few "cheat" meals. We can eat cake and fast food at some point but it's best to get where we want to be before we even think about this.

Step two – Plan your exercise routine

Your exercise routine is going to be the next step. Decide how you want to train. Pick one of the ready-made routines or use a blank routine card to create your own. You can change your workout method from week to week, or even daily. For example, you could train with bodyweight on Monday, barbells on Wednesday and perform a multi workout circuit on Friday. If, however, you are unfamiliar with certain exercises, or are a beginner it's probably best if you keep it simple and follow a single routine for the week.

Step three – Execute and stay consistent

Each week, you can reassess your diet or exercise. Make a new shopping list and plan new meals if you are not happy with something, but remember to follow the principals of portion size and quality nutrition if you make changes. Exercise can be changed too. If you feel you are not challenged enough, try increasing the workload by adding more sets, reps or resistance to exercises.

It really is this simple

You could explore different approaches to diet and follow a fasting method, a keto, paleo, raw, juice, Mediterranean, south beach, flexitarian, macrobiotic (the list goes on) diet and if it's something that works for you, great! But when you step back and look at most diet ideas, they are all actually rooted in the same simple concept that this book offers which is:

Nutritious foods eaten in the right quantities

Exercising regularly with resistance training, using compound movements and targeting every major muscle group is the next piece of the puzzle. If we train with moderate to high intensity, 3 -5 times per week, we have the puzzle solved.

Question and analyse the foods you choose to have as part of your diet, are they nutritious, do they support your goal? Make sure you are not over eating. Learn and master the exercise movements that you have in your workout routine, can you feel the target muscle group working? Check your exercise form if you can't. Do you have the right intensity in your workouts? Make sure you are pushing yourself but never sacrifice exercise form for more resistance.

The above paragraphs sum up this entire guide. It does not have to be complicated or overwhelming to get in shape. Learning anything new takes time, this includes exercise techniques and nutrition. The exercise and diet information in this book are the basics, and the basics, done well is all you need for body composition change. They are transferable skills that can be used for the rest of your life, whichever fitness path you choose to go down.

Exercise routine cards

Exercise routines can be documented on program cards. This is part of the planning phase and an excellent way to keep track of things from week to week.

I have designed the cards in this book to show which muscle group is being worked, which exercise is being performed, the sets and reps planned, and the workout schedule.

Many people will only need a single workout card for the six week duration. But it is possible to tweak or change your workout routine as you progress. As mentioned earlier, fitness progression is very rarely linear. It may be that after several weeks you find the workouts less challenging, so you will need to upgrade your routine by adding more reps, sets, exercises or even workouts per week. With an exercise card such as this one, you can easily keep track of this and plan ahead.

In my experience, it's very rewarding to look back at old exercise cards to remind us how far we have come. This can be a great boost to motivation.

Here's a visual explanation of an exercise card:

EXERCISE CARD			

ROUTINE #	1	MY ROUTINE		

You can name your routine and add a number if you wish to upgrade after several weeks.

MUSCLE GROUP	EXERCISE	SETS	REPS
CHEST	CHEST PRESS WITH DUMBBELLS	3	12
BACK	ROW WITH DUMBBELLS	3	12
LEGS	SQUATS WITH DUMBBELLS	3	12
BICEPS	BICEP CURL WITH DUMBBELLS	3	12
SHOULDERS	SHOULDER PRESS WITH DUMBBELLS	3	12
TRICEPS	TRICEP EXTENSIONS WITH DUMBBELLS	3	12
ABS	CRUNCHES	3	12

This is your workout, including the muscle groups worked, exercises planned, and sets and reps to be performed.

WEEKS	MON	TUE	WED	THURS	FRI	SAT	SUN
1	*		*		*		
2	*		*		*		
3	*		*		*		
4	*		*		*		*
5	*		*		*		*
6	*		*		*		*

This is the schedule for your workouts. The routine will occur on days marked with an asterisk (*). We can gradually increase the frequency of workouts each week.

If you plan on creating your own workouts, the blank cards at the back of the book can be printed off or copied for personal use. I always recommend that readers use these cards and create their own plan as this way, the workouts can be tailored to your needs. There are a lot of possibilities for variation; we can add extra exercises for weaker muscle groups, change exercises to suite the equipment we have, change exercises to suite our abilities etc.

I'm always happy to take a look at a routine that has been created and offer solutions or ideas, so if you go down this route and have questions, give me a shout.

Plan your exercise routine

Before you start training with resistance, rather than just picking up one of the exercise routine cards a few minutes before your workout, it's far better to have a plan well in advance.

This is a step that's too often overlooked in my experience. Like the diet side of things, we want to make sure we set ourselves up for success from the beginning. There are a few things we need to have in place before committing to a routine and making a start.

It is possible that ideas may change, but having something solid to work from at the beginning will make any later alterations easier to transition to. Also, like the diet advice, this is almost never a straightforward route, but if we consider the following points when planning our exercise routines, it will be our best guess and therefore, our best possible start.

Planning a full six weeks ahead would be great, but it may take a bit more work upfront, not to mention unforeseen circumstances that may change this. Planning a week ahead gives you the chance to tweak the following week once you get there. It might be that you find your current week of training doesn't challenge you enough, so you can make changes to your plan for the following week.

Step one

There are several training methods highlighted in this book. Standard "sets and reps" training, "circuit training" and "split training". You should decide which style you would like to use.

If you are new to resistance exercise, I would advise starting with a standard sets and reps style of exercise. This gives you chance to learn the exercise movements, become more confident, and find your strengths weaknesses and your effective workload.

If you are confident that you are performing the exercises correctly and effectively with the right workload, you can consider circuit training.

If you wish to progress to split training, you can do so with either a standard sets and reps training style, or even circuit training.

Step two

Most people lead busy lives and have commitments. If we truly want results from an exercise routine, it is a necessity that we find time to weave training sessions into our existing daily routines. So the first step is to sort this out. For the purpose of this guide, we need to train at a bare minimum of three times per week, preferably on non-consecutive days to sufficiently challenge ourselves for fitness progression.

Find times that are most convenient for you. Make a note of the days and times you plan to train on as you will need to fill them in on your routine card.

Step three

Once you have decided on your training style, find an appropriate card to use. There are many options to choose from in this guide. You could select one of the pre-made routine cards, or create your own from one of the blank options at the back of the book.

If you have chosen to create your own routine using multi workouts, make sure you are familiar with the exercises before you start your first session.

Fill in the planned training days at the bottom and you are set!

If you are planning week by week rather than six week blocks, make sure that you plan in any upgrades or variations to your training before the next week starts.

If you need extra cards, I am happy to send PDF copies to you to print out. Just let me know which one you need. If you have questions about a particular routine that you have created, I am also happy give my thoughts and advice – Jim@jimshealthandmuscle.com

Exercise routines

For your convenience, this section offers program cards to follow based on the resistance exercise methods. These full body workouts using bodyweight, resistance bands, barbells and dumbbells can be copied or printed out for you to follow. If you are unsure of any exercise or need a refresher on how to perform it from time to time, you will find illustrated descriptions in section 2.

The muscle group and exercises have been filled in, but the sets, reps and workout schedule has been left blank. This is because the workload will be different for everyone.

Here are some guidelines:

- Beginners, a range of 10 – 12 reps of 3 – 4 sets
- Intermediate, a range of 12 – 15 reps of 4 sets
- Advanced, a range of 15 – 25 reps of 4 – 6 sets

Regardless of sets and rep range, we should always ensure that we are challenging ourselves with the resistance level but at the same time, we should never sacrifice good exercise form for an increased workload. While it is true that more resistance translates to more muscle, more resistance should be achieved over time with progressive overload. This point is often overlooked, especially if the trainer feels weak on certain movements.

The correct resistance level for you will be one that sees you struggling to maintain full range of motion and exercise form on your last few reps of the set.

The bodyweight routine

BODYWEIGHT TRAINING			

ROUTINE #			

MUSCLE GROUP	EXERCISE	SETS	REPS
CHEST	PUSH UPS		
BACK	BODYWEIGHT ROW		
LEGS	BODYWEIGHT SQUATS		
BICEPS	BODYWEIGHT BICEP CURL		
SHOULDERS	PIKE PUSH UPS		
TRICEPS	TRICEP PUSH UPS		
ABS	CRUNCHES		

WEEKS	MON	TUE	WED	THURS	FRI	SAT	SUN
1							
2							
3							
4							
5							
6							

The resistance band routine

RESISTANCE BAND TRAINING			

ROUTINE #			

MUSCLE GROUP	EXERCISE	SETS	REPS
CHEST	CHEST PRESS RESISTANCE WITH BANDS		
BACK	ROW WITH RESISTANCE BANDS		
LEGS	RESISTANCE BAND SQUATS		
BICEPS	RESISTANCE BAND BICEP CURL		
SHOULDERS	RESISTANCE BAND SHOULDER PRESS		
TRICEPS	OVERHEAD TRICEP EXTENSION		
ABS	CRUNCHES WITH RESISTANCE BAND		

WEEKS	MON	TUE	WED	THURS	FRI	SAT	SUN
1							
2							
3							
4							
5							
6							

The barbell routine

BARBELL TRAINING			

ROUTINE #			

MUSCLE GROUP	EXERCISE	SETS	REPS
CHEST	CHEST PRESS WITH BARBELL		
BACK	ROW WITH BARBELL		
LEGS	SQUATS WITH BARBELL		
BICEPS	BICEP CURL WITH BARBELL		
SHOULDERS	SHOULDER PRESS WITH BARBELL		
TRICEPS	TRICEP EXTENSIONS WITH BARBELL		
ABS	CRUNCHES		

WEEKS	MON	TUE	WED	THURS	FRI	SAT	SUN
1							
2							
3							
4							
5							
6							

The dumbbell routine

DUMBBELL TRAINING			

ROUTINE #		

MUSCLE GROUP	EXERCISE	SETS	REPS
CHEST	CHEST PRESS WITH DUMBBELLS		
BACK	ROW WITH DUMBBELLS		
LEGS	SQUATS WITH DUMBBELLS		
BICEPS	BICEP CURL WITH DUMBBELLS		
SHOULDERS	SHOULDER PRESS WITH DUMBBELLS		
TRICEPS	TRICEP EXTENSIONS WITH DUMBBELLS		
ABS	CRUNCHES		

WEEKS	MON	TUE	WED	THURS	FRI	SAT	SUN
1							
2							
3							
4							
5							
6							

Multi workouts

Training exclusively with one method may not suit some trainers. This could be down to the fact that they don't have the equipment or it could be down to the fact that the exercise choices are not suitable for them. Push ups for example is a bodyweight exercise and would feature in a full bodyweight workout routine, although there are ways to make a push up more beginner friendly, this exercise can be too challenging for many people, so a resistance band exercise that targets the same muscle group could be chosen instead. This would be resistance band chest press and it could take the place of push ups on a bodyweight workout routine.

Multi workout example 1

MULTI TRAINING			

ROUTINE #			

MUSCLE GROUP	EXERCISE	SETS	REPS
CHEST	PUSH UPS		
BACK	ROW WITH RESISTANCE BANDS		
LEGS	BODYWEIGHT SQUATS		
BICEPS	BICEP CURL WITH RESISTANCE BANDS		
SHOULDERS	SHOULDER PRESS RESISTANCE BANDS		
TRICEPS	TRICEP DIPS		
ABS	CRUNCHES		

WEEKS	MON	TUE	WED	THURS	FRI	SAT	SUN
1							
2							
3							
4							
5							
6							

Multi workout example 2

MULTI TRAINING			

ROUTINE #			

MUSCLE GROUP	EXERCISE	SETS	REPS
CHEST	CHEST PRESS RESISTANCE BAND		
BACK	BODYWEIGHT ROW		
LEGS	BODYWEIGHT SQUATS		
BICEPS	BICEP CURL WITH DUMBBELLS		
SHOULDERS	SHOULDER PRESS DUMBBELLS		
TRICEPS	OVERHEAD TRICEP EXTENSION		
ABS	CRUNCHES RESISTANCE BAND		

WEEKS	MON	TUE	WED	THURS	FRI	SAT	SUN
1							
2							
3							
4							
5							
6							

Multi workout example 3

MULTI TRAINING			

ROUTINE #			

MUSCLE GROUP	EXERCISE	SETS	REPS
CHEST	CHEST PRESS BARBELL		
BACK	ROW DUMBBELLS		
LEGS	SQUATS BARBELL		
BICEPS	BICEP CURL WITH DUMBBELLS		
SHOULDERS	SHOULDER PRESS BARBELL		
TRICEPS	TRICEP EXTENSION DUMBBELLS		
ABS	CRUNCHES RESISTANCE BAND		

WEEKS	MON	TUE	WED	THURS	FRI	SAT	SUN
1							
2							
3							
4							
5							
6							

47

Circuit training

Circuit training is an excellent fat burning and muscle toning workout method. This is because it involves sustained energy expenditure to perform a circuit and requires a higher level of cardio vascular fitness. As we are also mainly working with compound movements and performing full body workouts, it adds an even greater challenge to a circuit.

I would argue that circuit training is one of the most efficient training methods for the goal of muscle tone and fat loss for these reasons.

How circuit training works

Circuit training is a style of workout that sees the trainer performing several sets of multiple exercises back to back without a rest between movements.

This training style, however, is not for everyone. The most noteworthy of issues with circuit training is that it's not entirely beginner friendly. As the training is intense, fatigue can set in quickly, this can be too much for a trainer that has not already established a foundation in basic muscle development. As mentioned in the workload chapter, when muscles fatigue, exercise form can suffer. If this happens, we would not only lose focus on the working muscle group, but in the worst case, we open ourselves up to injury.

I think very highly of this style of workout as it not only puts trainers into a higher intensity workout by default, but it brings in the cardio vascular aspect of fitness that is not found in most other resistance style training. But it comes with a prerequisite. My advice for circuit training aspirants is to first develop the exercises that they wish to use in a circuit, once they are confident and comfortable with the exercise form, then these exercises can be added to a circuit.

This is what circuit training looks like:

Here's an example of a circuit training program card. This particular example is the bodyweight routine, changed into a circuit showing the same exercises in the same order:

BODYWEIGHT TRAINING			
CIRCUIT ROUTINE			
MUSCLE GROUP	EXERCISE	REPS	SETS
CHEST	PUSH UPS	12	
BACK	BODYWEIGHT ROW	12	
LEGS	BODYWEIGHT SQUATS	15	
BICEPS	BODYWEIGHT BICEP CURL	12	**3**
SHOULDERS	PIKE PUSH UPS	12	
TRICEPS	TRICEP PUSH UPS	12	
ABS	CRUNCHES	15	

WEEKS	MON	TUE	WED	THURS	FRI	SAT	SUN
1	*	*		*	*		
2	*	*		*	*		
3	*	*		*	*		
4	*	*	*	*	*		
5	*	*	*	*	*		
6	*	*	*	*	*		

As you can see, this is a complete six week plan for a full body circuit training routine. If we were to follow this, we would be training with only three sets per workout, but each set would consist of ninety reps split between seven exercises. We would also be training four times per week for the first three weeks and five times per week for the next three weeks.

The sets, reps and training days for this example routine have been filled in for explanation purposes, so, depending on the trainer, this can be adjusted for a better fit.

Circuit training is short, sharp but extremely effective. If you are a beginner, but would like to give this a go, it would certainly be worth putting in the time to develop the exercise form and a base of muscular strength for each movement that you would like to use. Your first six weeks could be the preparation and your next six weeks could be your first steps on your circuit training journey?

There are many ways to add circuit training into your existing routine. For example, I created a home workout for beginner's video course which takes the trainer through development of mind-set, basic compound movements and planning for fitness success. As this course is progressive, it steps up a gear each week and several weeks in we add circuit training to the last training session of the week.

This is something that can also be done when using this guide to plan your workouts.

The business man in me has a need to take this opportunity to mention more about this course for those who might be interested ☺

YourFitnessSuccess.com

For your convenience, the next few pages have each of the exclusive training types converted into circuits should you wish to use them for your main workouts or to mix them in with your existing routines.

The bodyweight circuit

BODYWEIGHT TRAINING			

CIRCUIT ROUTINE			

MUSCLE GROUP	EXERCISE	REPS	SETS
CHEST	PUSH UPS		
BACK	BODYWEIGHT ROW		
LEGS	BODYWEIGHT SQUATS		
BICEPS	BODYWEIGHT BICEP CURL		
SHOULDERS	PIKE PUSH UPS		
TRICEPS	TRICEP PUSH UPS		
ABS	CRUNCHES		

WEEKS	MON	TUE	WED	THURS	FRI	SAT	SUN
1							
2							
3							
4							
5							
6							

51

The resistance band circuit

RESISTANCE BAND TRAINING			

ROUTINE #			

MUSCLE GROUP	EXERCISE	REPS	SETS
CHEST	CHEST PRESS RESISTANCE WITH BANDS		
BACK	ROW WITH RESISTANCE BANDS		
LEGS	RESISTANCE BAND SQUATS		
BICEPS	RESISTANCE BAND BICEP CURL		
SHOULDERS	RESISTANCE BAND SHOULDER PRESS		
TRICEPS	OVERHEAD TRICEP EXTENSION		
ABS	CRUNCHES WITH RESISTANCE BAND		

WEEKS	MON	TUE	WED	THURS	FRI	SAT	SUN
1							
2							
3							
4							
5							
6							

52

The dumbbell circuit

DUMBBELL TRAINING			

ROUTINE #			

MUSCLE GROUP	EXERCISE	REPS	SETS
CHEST	CHEST PRESS WITH DUMBBELLS		
BACK	ROW WITH DUMBBELLS		
LEGS	SQUATS WITH DUMBBELLS		
BICEPS	BICEP CURL WITH DUMBBELLS		
SHOULDERS	SHOULDER PRESS WITH DUMBBELLS		
TRICEPS	TRICEP EXTENSIONS WITH DUMBBELLS		
ABS	CRUNCHES		

WEEKS	MON	TUE	WED	THURS	FRI	SAT	SUN
1							
2							
3							
4							
5							
6							

The barbell circuit

BARBELL CIRCUIT			

ROUTINE #			

MUSCLE GROUP	EXERCISE	REPS	SETS
CHEST	CHEST PRESS WITH BARBELL		
BACK	ROW WITH BARBELL		
LEGS	SQUATS WITH BARBELL		
BICEPS	BICEP CURL WITH BARBELL		
SHOULDERS	SHOULDER PRESS WITH BARBELL		
TRICEPS	TRICEP EXTENSIONS WITH BARBELL		
ABS	CRUNCHES		

WEEKS	MON	TUE	WED	THURS	FRI	SAT	SUN
1							
2							
3							
4							
5							
6							

Split training

The more you exercise, the better for energy expenditure, but, for muscle growth, we also need to rest. The routines in the previous chapter are single, full body workouts which means we should have rest days in order to recover. Split training gives us the opportunity to train most days as we focus on specific muscle groups per workout. I consider split training to be a more advanced training option as the workload per muscle group is increased.

If you get to a point where you are confident to add extra training days, your exercise form is good and you are recovering well between full body workouts, split training is a great option.

Rather than training a minimum of three times per week with a single routine, we increase to a minimum of four times per week using two separate routines. We would work from an "A" routine and a "B" routine consecutively. We work half our body during workout "A" and the other half during workout "B". On completion of a full week of training each muscle group would have been trained twice.

Here is an example of a 2 day split routine using resistance bands and bodyweight exercises:

EXERCISE CARD			

ROUTINE #		

MUSCLE GROUP	EXERCISE	SETS	REPS
	WORKOUT A		
CHEST	PUSH UPS		
CHEST	FLYS - RESISTANCE BANDS		
BACK	LAT PULL DOWN - RESISTANCE BANDS		
BACK	BODYWEIGHT ROW		
BICEPS	BICEP CURL - RESISTANCE BANDS		
	WORKOUT B		
TRICEPS	TRICEP PUSH UPS		
SHOULDERS	LATERAL RAISES - RESISTANCE BANDS		
SHOULDERS	PIKE PUSH UPS		
LEGS	BODYWEIGHT LUNGES		
LEGS	BODYWEIGHT SQUATS		

WEEKS	MON	TUE	WED	THURS	FRI	SAT	SUN
1	A	B		A	B		
2	A	B		A	B		
3	A	B		A	B		
4	A	B		A	B		
5	A	B		A	B		
6	A	B		A	B		

56

This split training routine sees us using a "multi workout" as we are performing exercises with bodyweight resistance and also exercise bands. In this example, we are training four times per week but hitting each major muscle group twice per week.

In the exercise session planner at the bottom, instead of simply marking a training day, we either enter "A" or "B" in this section ensuring that they are non-consecutive.

Workout "A"

Workout "A" targets chest, back and biceps.

Workout "B"

Workout "B" targets triceps, shoulders and legs

Split training sessions can be more intensive as there is longer rest between challenging certain body parts. This means we can add extra exercises to each muscle group.

When working with multiple exercises for a single muscle group, I would advise that these exercises are sequential. For example, if we use a chest press (push up) and a pec fly movement in the same workout, once we have completed every set of push ups (targeting the chest muscles), our next exercise would also be for chest. In this example, it would be "flys with resistance bands".

As you can see from the example, this is shown in the list of exercises.

Sets and rep range

I consider split training to be a more advanced option, so would suggest that the sets and reps are higher than beginner values:

4 sets of 12 -15 reps with moderate to high intensity is the goal.

Training days

The days marked for training on the example are ideal as there is a single rest day after the body has been fully worked and double rest days after the body has had its second full workout. This should give the intermediate to advanced trainer adequate time to recover before the next week of training.

Section 2

The Exercises

Most exercises in this section are compound movements. Compound exercises are those that involve more than one muscle group to complete a single rep. When compared to isolation exercises, compound movements are far superior for the goal of fat loss and muscle tone as more muscle groups are challenged per rep which means more energy is expended and due to the nature of these movements, it is usually possible to use more resistance. More resistance means gains in strength too.

Chest press, row movements, squats and shoulder press are excellent compound exercises and are used as the foundation for every program card featured in this guide. Here's a breakdown of the muscle groups used when each of these movements is performed.

This is useful to know as mind muscle connection significantly enhances our performance and progress. So when exercising make a conscious effort to fully engage the intended muscle group. If you are working through a chest press exercise for example, but you feel other muscle groups such as your shoulders working, you may need to revisit the exercise description.

Chest press

When performing any chest press movement, the main muscles being worked are the chest or "pecs". As this is a compound movement, the triceps and front deltoids are also used as synergists.

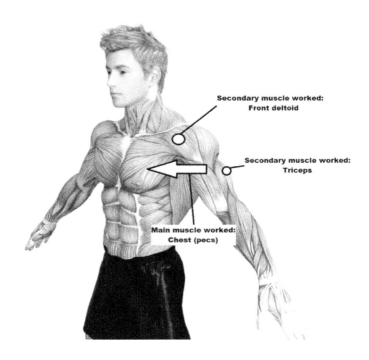

Secondary muscle worked:
Front deltoid

Secondary muscle worked:
Triceps

Main muscle worked:
Chest (pecs)

Row

A rowing movement is a compound movement. The main muscles being worked are the back or "lats". Other muscles such as the biceps, rear shoulder and trapezius muscles are also worked during this movement.

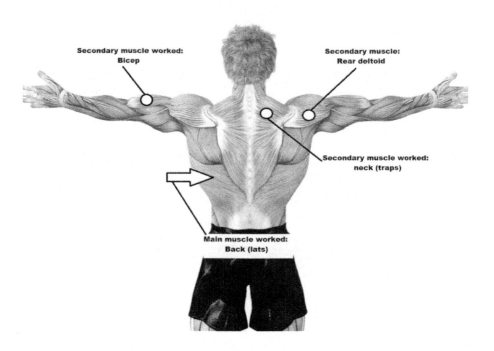

Secondary muscle worked:
Bicep

Secondary muscle:
Rear deltoid

Secondary muscle worked:
neck (traps)

Main muscle worked:
Back (lats)

Squat

The squat is a big compound movement that mainly targets the front, upper leg muscles or "quads". Muscles that are also involved in a squat movement are the glutes, hamstrings and lower back.

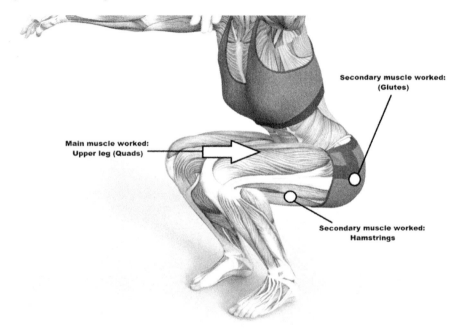

Secondary muscle worked: (Glutes)

Main muscle worked: Upper leg (Quads)

Secondary muscle worked: Hamstrings

Shoulder press

When performing a shoulder press movement, all three heads of the shoulders or "delts" are engaged. These are the front, lateral and rear. As this is a compound movement, there are other muscle groups that work in synergy. These are the traps, chest and biceps.

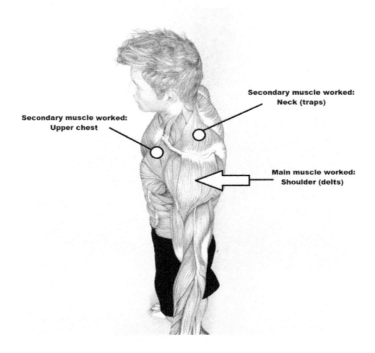

Secondary muscle worked:
Neck (traps)

Secondary muscle worked:
Upper chest

Main muscle worked:
Shoulder (delts)

Bicep curl, tricep extension, abdominal exercises

Although bicep curl, tricep extension and crunches (abdominal exercises) are not considered compound exercises, they are included in this guide to offer a direct workload to these muscle groups to give a more complete workout

Chest

Push ups

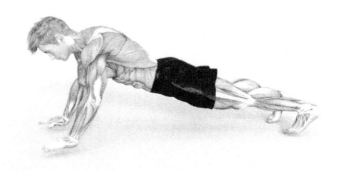

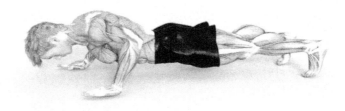

Description:

- Take a position so your palms and toes are in contact with the floor
- Palms should be in line with your mid chest and about shoulder width apart
- Arms should be straight with a slight bend in the elbows
- Back should be flat and head in a neutral position
- As you inhale, lower your upper body towards the floor by bending at the elbows, insuring your elbows stay close to your sides rather than flaring out
- Once you feel a suitable stretch across your chest, or your noes grazes the floor, exhale and return to the start position
- This completes one rep

Extra info:

Full push ups can be challenging for some trainers. It is possible to work up to this by performing the same movement with your knees in contact with the floor rather than your toes. It is also less challenging to perform the movement with your hands on an elevated surface, such as a workout bench

Flys with resistance bands

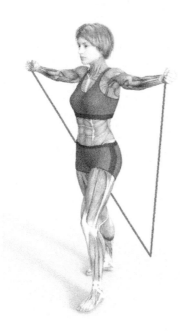 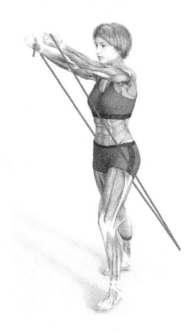

Description:

- Select an appropriate resistance band for your fitness level. Attach a door anchor to secure the band to the bottom of a door. Ensure that there are even lengths of band either side of the anchor point
- Attach hand stirrups to either end of the band as an optional step
- Grip both ends of the band and raise your arms out to your sides with your back to the anchor point. Palms should be facing forward
- With your arms straight out to your sides and parallel to the floor, step forward until you feel resistance on the band
- As you exhale, bring your palms together and slightly upwards across the front of your body. Arms should remain straight with a slight bend in the elbows
- Once you reach the top of movement, inhale and return to the start position. This completes one rep

Extra info:

This movement is an isolation exercise for the chest and for the purpose of this guide; it should be used in addition to a chest press movement rather than a substitute. Variations to this exercise can be to attach the anchor point to the top of the door rather than the bottom. When doing this, instead of bringing the palms together and slightly upwards, bring them together and slightly downwards.

Chest press with resistance band

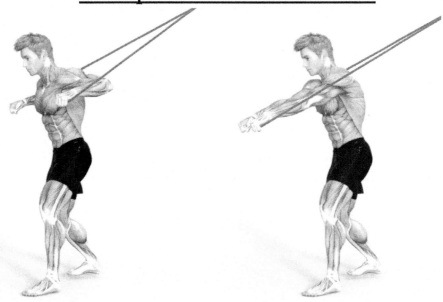

Description:

- Select an appropriate resistance band for your fitness level. Attach a door anchor to secure the band to the top of a door. Ensure that there are even lengths of band either side of the anchor point
- Attach hand stirrups to either end of the band as an optional step
- Grip both ends of the band and raise your arms so your fists are in line with your mid chest. Palms should be facing down
- Hinge at the hips slightly and take a step forward until your feel tension on the band
- As you exhale, push your fists forward and slightly downward into the centre line of your body by straightening your arms
- Once your fists meet at your centre line, inhale and return to the start position

Extra info:

The variation of this exercise movement is to attach the door anchor to the bottom of the door. When doing this, instead of pushing your fists forward and slightly down, you should push your fists forward and slightly upwards when performing the movement.

Chest press with dumbbells

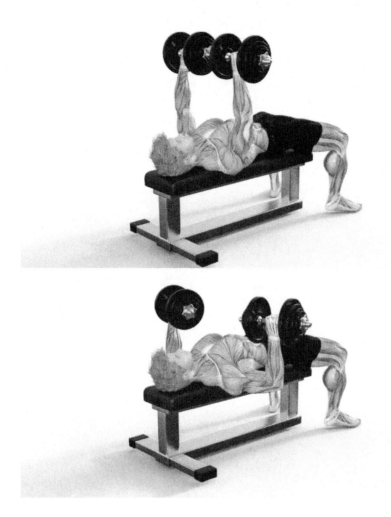

Description:

- A flat workout bench is required for this exercise
- Select a set of dumbbells appropriate for your set, sit on the bench resting them on your quads
- As you lie on the bench, bring the dumbbells towards your chest
- Straighten your arms directly above your mid chest, palms facing towards your lower body

- As you inhale, lower the dumbbells towards your chest by bending at the elbows and extending the shoulder
- Once you feel a suitable stretch across your chest, this is the top of movement. At this point, as you exhale, return to the start position

Extra info:

During this movement, it's important that the dumbbells do not drift either inwards or outwards. A good thing to keep in mind is that the weight should always run in a direct line through the length of your forearm to the floor. If this is a new exercise, it may take some practice, but once this is perfected, the movement will feel more stable.

Chest press with a barbell

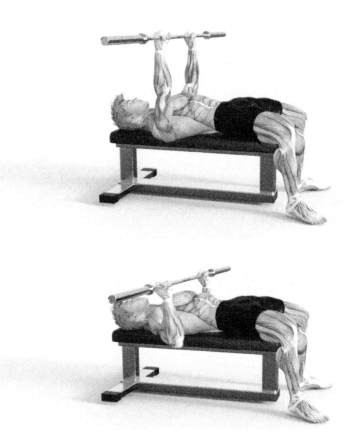

Description:

- A flat workout bench is required for this exercise. Depending on your set up and resistance level used, you may also need a rack for the barbell
- Lie flat on the bench. Grip the bar so your hands are about shoulder width apart
- Lift the bar away from the rack and with straight (elbows slightly bent) hold the bar above the line of your mid chest.

- As you inhale, lower the bar towards your mid chest by bending at the elbows
- Once you feel the stretch across your chest you have reached the top of movement, exhale as you return to the start position

Extra info:

Often, "the top of movement" will be the point where the barbell grazes the mid chest, but for some who have less flexibility, it may be higher than this. It is important to achieve a full range of motion with any exercise, but always be aware of over extending relative to your current flexibility level. Keep the negative movement slow and controlled, bigger range of motion can be an ongoing goal.

Back

Bodyweight row

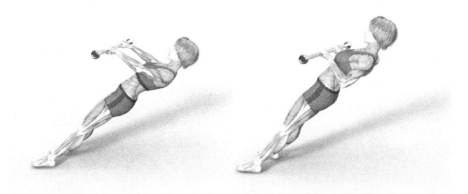

Description:

- You will need a solid platform with space underneath for your body. Workout equipment such as dips bars or a pull up bar attached to a lower point in a doorway can be used for this.
- Grip the bar so your hands are about shoulder width apart, palms facing down
- Position yourself underneath it by planting your feet firmly on the floor. You will need to take the weight of your body by holding onto the bar while you get into position
- Once the bar is in line with your mid chest, straighten your arms, keep your back flat and head in a neutral position
- As you exhale, pull your upper body towards the bar by bending your elbows and pulling your shoulders back. Keep your elbows close you your body throughout this movement
- Once your chest grazes the bar, as you exhale, return to the start position

Extra info:

Although it is best to do this exercise with specialist equipment, there are a number of ways it can be improvised (a solid bar across two chairs being one). But if you do improvise a set up for this, make sure it is solid. A bar rolling off its standing, or even breaking can cause injuries. The risk is not worth taking.

This exercise can be made incrementally more challenging by changing the angle of the start position. The lower the bar, or the more acute the angle from the back of your body to the floor, the more advanced the exercise becomes. Beginners can perform this exercise from a near standing position while advanced trainers can perform the exercise from close to a lying position.

Row with resistance band

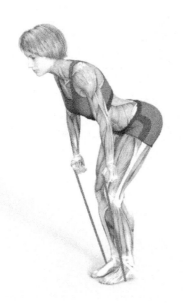 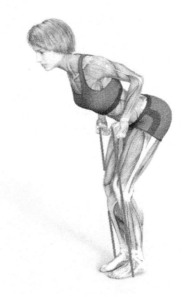

Description:

- Select an exercise band, grip the ends, palms facing inwards and stand in the middle of the band with both feet ensuring there are equal lengths either side of your feet
- Bend your knees slightly and hinge at the hips to assume a slightly forward leaning position
- Ensure that your upper back is flat, head in a neutral position and arms straight placing your fists near your knees
- At this point you may need to adjust your grip on the band so there is tension. Simply grip the band at a closer point to your feet
- As you exhale, pull your fists towards your navel. As you do this, keep your elbows close to the sides of your body
- Once you are at the top of movement, as you inhale, return to the start position

Extra info:

Attaching the stirrups to an exercise band for this exercise will probably not work. Most resistance bands have a generous length to them and stirrups are designed to be attached to the ends. This movement, however, almost always requires the trainer to grip the band closer to the mid-point. It is normal to have excess resistance band trailing. If this is distracting, it can be wrapped around the hands as you get into the start position.

Row with dumbbells

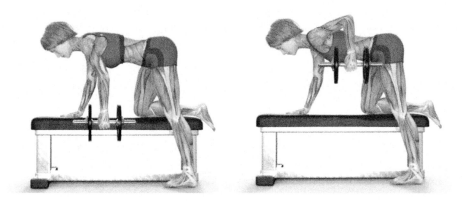

Description:

- A workout bench or similar solid platform is needed for this exercise.
- Select a single dumbbell appropriate for your fitness level and grip it in your left hand
- Kneel on the bench with your right knee. Plant your left on the floor
- Hinge at the hips to place your right hand on the bench.
- At this point, your back should be flat, head in a neutral position and the dumbbell should be held in position with a straight arm, elbow slightly bent
- As you exhale, pull the dumbbell towards your navel. Your elbow should graze the side of your body and reach a position that is higher than your back
- Once at the top of movement, as you inhale, return to the start position
- Once the set is complete, repeat the set on the other side. (Dumbbell in the right hand, left knee and hand on the bench)

Extra info:

This exercise can be performed without a specialised workout bench. Two chairs, one for the knee and one for the hand can be used, but there is a risk of the chairs slipping if they are not attached to the floor. It is possible to use a sofa for this exercise, but I would advise that a solid surface without thick cushioning is much more appropriate.

Finally, I consider this exercise to be an advanced choice as it does require a good "mind-muscle" connection and a higher amount of concentration than other exercises.

Row with a barbell

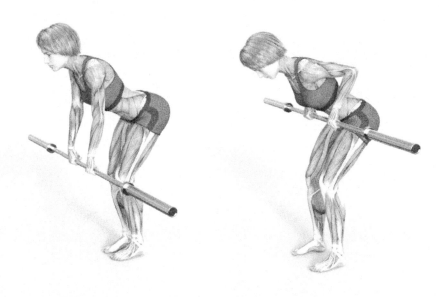

Description:

- Hold a barbell with an overhand grip, hands about shoulder width apart
- Bend your knees slightly and hinge at the hips to position your upper body so it's at about a forty-five degrees to the floor
- Keep your back flat and head in a neutral position
- Your arms should be straight with a slight bend in the elbows to position the bar close to your upper legs
- As you exhale, pull the bar towards your navel. Your elbows should not flare out and should move above your back
- Once at the top of movement, as you inhale, return to the start position

Extra info:

With bent over row movements using free weights, it's easy to lose concentration and change the angle of the upper body during the set, so be aware of this. If the angle changes too much and the upper body moves to a more upright position, the workload on the latissimus dorsi (back muscles) will transfer to the rear shoulder and trap muscles.

Legs

Bodyweight squats

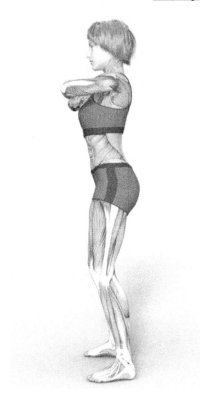
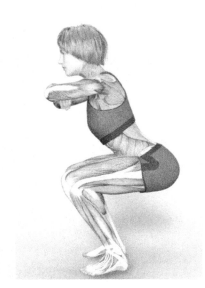

Description:

- Stand with your feet just past shoulder width apart, keep your head in a neutral position and maintain a flat back
- Fold your arms across your body at shoulder height, ensuring they are parallel to the floor
- As you inhale, bend at the knees to lower your upper body towards the floor
- Keep your back flat and arms in the start position throughout the movement
- As you exhale, push through your heels to straighten your legs again. You should not lock your knees at the top of movement to keep the tension on your quads
- This completes one rep

Extra info:

Squat movements are excellent lower body exercises, but they can take some practice. Common issues with the ability to perform a good squat are weaknesses or inflexibility of certain muscle groups involved. This can also lead to a lack of confidence in the movement. The best way to develop all muscle groups is to keep practicing squats. If there is a confidence issue, meaning you feel you may fall backwards when squatting, a low chair or bench can be placed underneath the glutes. From my experience, this can make all the difference from a lack of confidence standpoint.

Bodyweight lunges

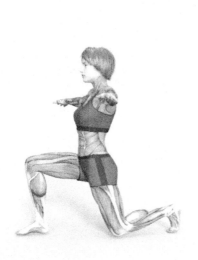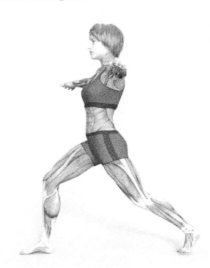

Description:

- Kneel so that your left knee and toes of your left foot contact the floor
- The foot of your right leg should be placed flat on the floor. There should be a right angle between the back of your right upper and lower leg
- Keep your back flat and head in a neutral position
- For balance, lift your arms out to your sides
- As you exhale, push through the centre of your right foot and toes of your left foot in equal measure. This will straighten your legs by bending at the knee
- Once at the top of movement, inhale and return to the start position
- Once you complete the set, mirror the process and repeat it on the opposite leg

Extra info:

Between reps, when "returning to the start position", you should not rest your knee on the floor. Pause briefly a small distance before contact. This will keep tension on the working muscles and deliver more value from the set.

Squats with resistance band

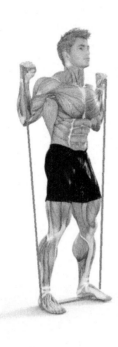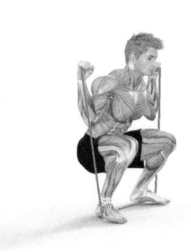

Description:

- Select a resistance band appropriate for your fitness level and attach hand stirrups if you have them
- Hold the stirrups in your hands and step on the band so it runs through the mid-point of the soles of your feet. Your feet should be about shoulder width apart. Ensure you have equal lengths of band either side
- Stand straight with a flat back, head in a neutral position. Raise your fists so your palms are facing forward and are in line with your shoulders
- As you inhale, bend at the knees to lower your upper body towards the floor
- Keep your back flat and fists as per the start position
- As you exhale, push through your heels to straighten your legs again. You should not lock your knees at the top of movement to keep the tension on your quads
- This completes one rep

Extra info:

For some more advanced trainers, resistance band squats will require more resistance than a single band gives in order to reach an appropriate workload or intensity level. This can be achieved by attaching multiple resistance bands to the stirrups. If you need to do this, ensure that all resistance bands used are the same length. This is usually the case if all bands are used from the same set.

Squats with dumbbells

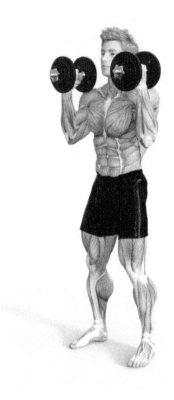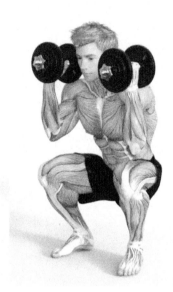

Description:

- Select a set of dumbbells appropriate for your fitness level
- Stand straight and hold the dumbbells with a hammer type grip (Palms facing towards the mid-line of your body
- Bend your elbows and twist through the shoulders to rest the dumbbells on your shoulders
- Stand with your feet just past shoulder width apart, knees slightly bent
- As you inhale, lower your upper body by bending at the knees until your upper legs are at least parallel with the floor
- Throughout the movement, keep your back flat and head in a neutral position

94

- Once at the top of movement, as you exhale, return to the start position. You should push through the middle or slightly towards the heels of your feet to do this
- On returning to the start position, this is one rep

Extra info:

There are a few variations of grip that can be used for dumbbell squats. A single dumbbell can be used by holding the weight close to the chest. This exercise can also be performed with palms facing forward, but in my opinion, the description used in this book is the best as the dumbbells are not only secure, but the resistance is in such a position that it takes strain away from the wrists and forearm muscles, allowing for greater concentration on the exercise overall.

Squats with a barbell

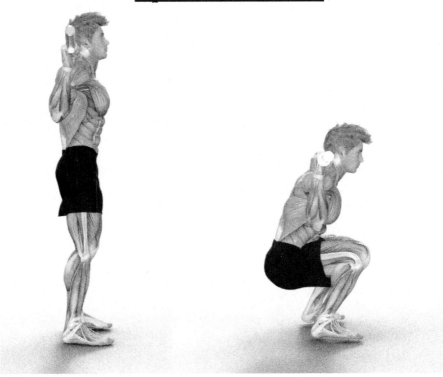

Description:

- Select a barbell appropriate for your fitness level. Depending on the amount of weight used, you may need a rack for this exercise
- Stand underneath a racked barbell and position the centre knurl in the middle of your traps
- Grip the barbell at the same distance from the centre either side, palms facing forward
- Maintaining a flat back and neutral head position, stand up to take the weight on your shoulders
- Your feet should be slightly wider than shoulder width apart
- As you inhale, lower your upper body by bending at the knees until your upper legs are at least parallel with the floor
- Throughout the movement, keep your back flat and head in a neutral position

96

- Once at the top of movement, as you exhale, return to the start position. You should push through the middle or slightly towards the heels of your feet to do this
- On returning to the start position, this is one rep

Extra info:

As it is with all squatting exercises, before attempting any resistance with a barbell, you should be comfortable with bodyweight squats. If you are new to squats but plan on using a barbell later in your training, you can use a broom handle or light wooden bar in order to become familiar with the positioning and general feel of a barbell on your shoulders.

Shoulders

Pike push ups

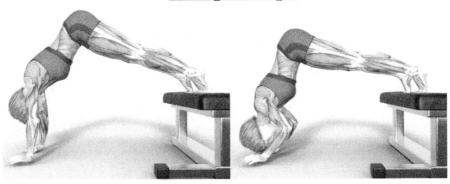

Description:

- You will need a workout bench or other solid platform to work from
- Assume a push up position and place your toes on your workout bench
- Once your body is in an incline push up position, walk your hands closer to the bench as you hinge at the hips
- Once you have reached an appropriate angle for your fitness level, ensure your back is flat, legs are straight, arms are straight with a slight bend at the elbows
- Your hands should be spaced just past shoulder width apart
- As you inhale, bend at the elbows to lower your upper body towards the floor
- Once your forehead is about to make contact with the floor, exhale and return to the start position by straightening your arms
- Once at the start position, this completes one rep

Extra info:

This is an advanced exercise and should only be performed by trainers that have a good foundation of strength training. Although this is predominantly a shoulder press exercise, many other muscle groups are challenged during the movement.

The closer to the bench that the trainer walks their hands in the set up phase of this movement, the more concentrated the shoulder exercise will be. If range of movement is not sufficient for the trainer, push up bars can be used to gain extra depth.

Shoulder press with resistance band

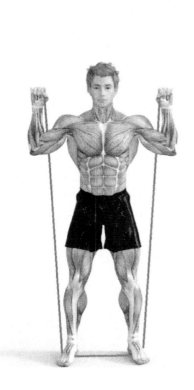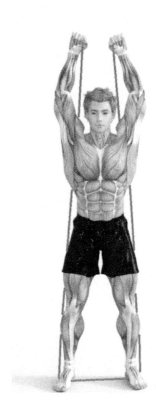

Description:

- Select an exercise band appropriate for your fitness level and attach the hand stirrups
- Stand in the middle of the band with both feet ensuring there are even lengths of band either side
- Grip the stirrups and stand up straight, back flat, knees slightly bent and head in a neutral position
- Hold the stirrups palms facing forward and in line with your chin. Your hands should also be in line with your shoulders
- As you exhale, push your fists directly above your head, bringing them closer together as you progress through the movement

- Once your arms are almost straight and your fists are about to touch, this is the top of movement
- Exhale and return to the start position to complete one rep

Extra info:

Limited flexibility through the shoulders can make this difficult. If the start and top of movement positions are challenging, the exercise can still be performed, but to get the most benefit, the trainer should look at improving flexibility in this area. Limited shoulder mobility on this exercise can lead to a development of the front deltoid and neglect the rear, causing more imbalances.

You can choose to stand with one foot on the band. To do, set up as per the description but take a step forward with one foot. This foot should be placed in the middle of the band.

Shoulder press with dumbbells

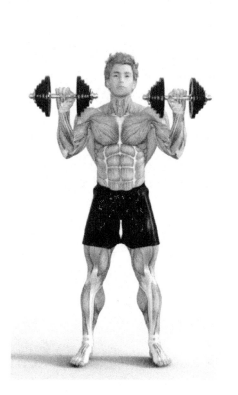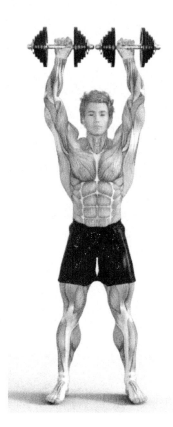

Description:

- Select a set of dumbbells that are appropriate for your fitness level
- Grip the dumbbells and stand up straight, back flat, knees slightly bent and head in a neutral position
- Hold the dumbbells palms facing forward and in line with your chin. Your hands should also be in line with your shoulders
- As you exhale, push your fists directly above your head, bringing them closer together as you progress through the movement
- Once your arms are almost straight and dumbbells are about to touch, this is the top of movement
- Exhale and return to the start position to complete one rep

Extra info:

When performing the movement with dumbbells, doing so in front of a mirror is helpful. The bars or the dumbbells should always remain parallel with the floor. If they are angled either to the left or right, the weight distribution will also shift this way. This can cause undue pressure on the elbows and shoulders whilst also diluting the workload in the deltoids.

Shoulder press with barbell

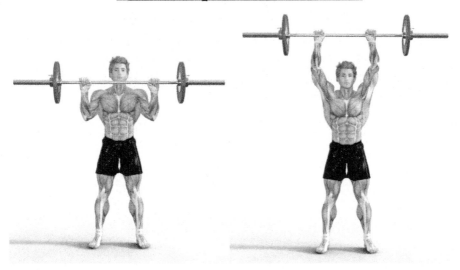

Description:

- Choose a barbell that is appropriate for your fitness level. Ideally, this bar will be set on a rack, just below shoulder height.
- Stand in front of the racked bar and grip it about a hands span past shoulder width making sure your body is in the centre of the bar
- Keep your knees slightly bent, back flat and head in a neutral position after you un rack the bar to take the weight
- As you exhale, push the bar directly above your head until just before your elbows are about to lock
- Once at the top of movement, slowly return to the start position as you inhale. This completes one rep
- Once the set is complete, re rack the bar

Extra info:

A common issue with this exercise is to hyperextend through the lower back (hips go forward and upper body moves backwards). Be aware of this position. The load should run down, through the mid line of your body.

Foot spacing can be changed depending on the trainer. One foot forward is possible, but through experience, I have noticed this can lead to an imbalance of shoulder strength from one side to the other. If you do decide to do this, alternate between your forward placed foot each set.

Standing with your feet close together adds more challenge to the exercise as stabiliser muscles are engaged a lot more.

Biceps

Bodyweight bicep curl

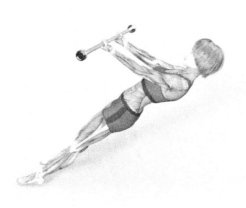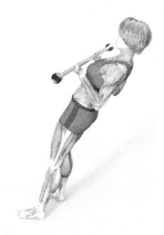

Description:

- Set up a pull up bar between a door at mid abdominal height. Alternatively, you can use a dips bar or similar sturdy platform
- Take an underhand grip (Palms facing up) on the bar so your hands are shoulder width apart
- Position your lower body underneath the bar as you take your body weight
- Straighten your arms to put them out in front of you until your elbows are about to lock
- Ensure the full posterior of your body has a flat alignment
- As you exhale, pull your upper towards the bar by bending at the elbows and pulling your shoulders back
- Ensure the insides of your arms stay close to the sides of your upper body (don't flare your elbows outwards)
- Once at the top of movement, as you inhale, return to the start position. This completes one rep

Extra info:

This is an advance exercise and requires a good foundation of muscle strength to perform correctly. Moving the bar higher will make the exercise less challenging, this can be worthwhile if you are new to the exercise.

For advanced trainers using this exercise, the bar can be lower. This will dictate leg position and may require a bend in the knees. Keeping the back flat above the knees, using an underhand grip and keeping the elbows close to the body during the movement are all key ingredients to making this exercise target the biceps.

Bicep curl with resistance band

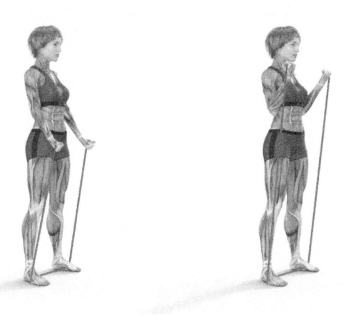

Description:

- Select a resistance band that's appropriate for your fitness level. Attaching the stirrups is optional
- Stand in the middle of the band ensuring there are even lengths either side
- Hold the ends of the band with straight arms, palms facing forward
- Elbows should be slightly bent and upper arms should be by your sides but slightly forward of the front of your body
- Keep your knees slightly bent, back flat, head in a neutral position
- Keeping your upper arms fixed in the start position, exhale as you bend your elbows to bring your palms towards the fronts of your shoulders
- Ensure that your palms are facing your shoulders at the top of movement (don't rotate them inwards for this version of bicep curls)
- Once at the top of movement, exhale as you return to the start position
- This completes one rep

Extra info:

Choosing to attach the stirrups will depend on the length of your bands. Longer bands may not have enough tension with the stirrups attached to make this an effective exercise. At the start position, simply gripping the band at the point that there is tension is usually the best approach here. Excess band can be wrapped around your hands if it is a distraction.

Bicep curl with dumbbells

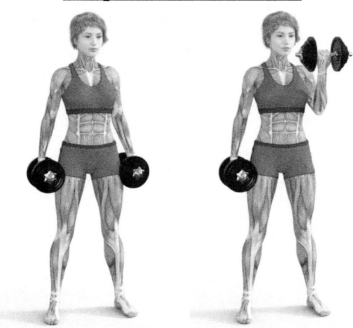

Description:

- Select a set of dumbbells that are appropriate for your fitness level.
- Stand up straight, knees slightly bent, feet about shoulder width apart, and head in a neutral position whilst holding the dumbbells by your sides, palms facing inwards
- Although straight, your arms should have a slight bend at the elbows
- As you exhale rotate your shoulder slightly to place your upper arm slightly in front of your body. Once in this position, the shoulder stops moving
- Bend at the elbow to bring the dumbbell towards your shoulder. As you progress through the movement, twist your palm outwards
- Once at the top of movement, your palm should be facing your shoulder and bicep should be contracted
- At this point, inhale and return to the start position and repeat on the opposite arm. Once the movement has been completed on the opposite arm, this completes one rep

Extra info:

The industry name for this exercise is "supination curl". It differs from other bicep curls in this guide in that it starts as a "hammer movement" (palm facing your mid line). This version of a bicep curl has a focus on the long head of the bicep along with forearm muscles.

Bicep curls with dumbbells can be performed in a seated position. Some trainers prefer this as they find it offers an opportunity for more focus to the muscle group.

Bicep curl with a barbell

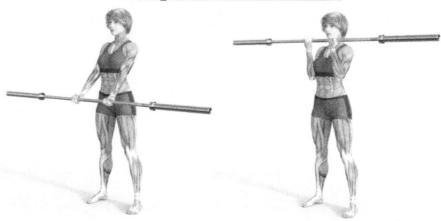

Description:

- Select a barbell with the appropriate resistance for your fitness level
- Hold the bar with an underhand grip (palms facing upwards). Hands should be about shoulder width apart and set so there are even lengths either side of the bar
- Stand upright with a slight bend in the knees, back flat and head in a neutral position
- Straighten your arms until there is only a slight bend in the elbows and pull your shoulders slightly backwards
- The barbell should be at about waist height at the start position
- As you exhale, bend at the elbows to bring the bar towards your upper body
- Once your biceps reach maximum contraction, this is the top of movement.
- At this point, inhale as you return to the start position. This completes one rep

Extra info:

This is an excellent exercise for bicep strength and growth, but the exercise form needed needs to be strict. A weighted bar can act as a pendulum during this movement and dilute the training effect significantly, so it's important to keep a flat back and pause at the end of each rep to make every rep count.

Some trainers benefit from performing this exercise with full back contact against a solid wall to ensure maximum workload on the biceps by negating any unnecessary movement.

Triceps

Tricep dips

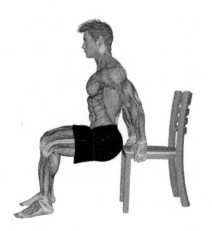 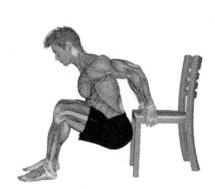

Description:

- You will need a workout bench or a sturdy chair
- Take the weight of your body by holding onto the bench to leave your upper body suspended in front of the bench
- Your feet should be firmly planted on the floor with your knees bent
- Keep your back flat and head in a neutral position
- As you inhale, lower your upper body by bending at the elbows. You should only lower to the point where you feel the stretch on your triceps
- As you lower allow your elbows to flare out naturally, but not too much
- Once at the top of movement, as you exhale, push through your palms to straighten your arms and return to the start position
- This completes one rep

Extra info:

This is an exercise that does not suit everyone. Some instructors will advise that you keep your elbows pushed back, not allowing them to flare out. I advise otherwise, this is why; this exercise can put a lot of strain on the shoulder and forcing the elbows towards the midline increases the strain.

Tricep dips are a good exercise for the back of the arms, but if you find this uncomfortable, it may be worth finding an alternative.

Overhead tricep extension

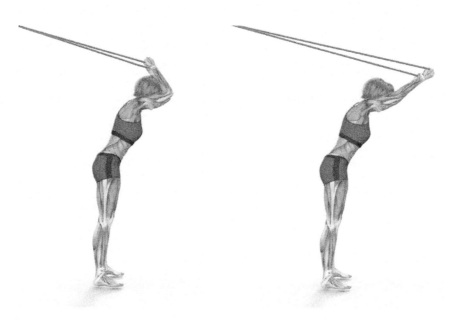

Description:

- Select a resistance band that's appropriate for your fitness level. Attach a door anchor at the top of a door or anchor above head height.
- Ensure you have even lengths of band either side of the anchor point
- Stand with your back to the anchor point and a few steps away. Grip the ends of the band in each hand, palms facing inwards
- Raise hinge at the hips keeping your back flat and knees slightly bent to put your upper body at a slight angle. You may want to place one foot forward for balance
- Raise your arms so your upper arms are above parallel with the floor and bend at the elbows so your fists are slightly behind your head
- If there is no tension on the band at this point, take a step or two forward
- As you exhale, bend at the elbows to straighten your arms. Your upper arms should remain fixed
- Once your arms are straight, this is the top of movement and you can inhale and return to the start position. This completes one rep

Extra info:

A common issue with this exercise is that during the set, the upper arms can drop. This causes a significant dilution of workload to the triceps. After each set, it's worth making a conscious effort to reset the start position, especially where the position of the upper arms are concerned.

Tricep extension with dumbbell

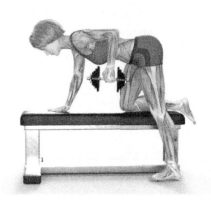 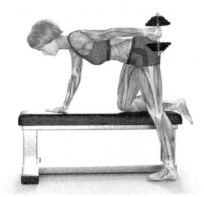

Description:

- A workout bench or similar solid platform is needed for this exercise.
- Select a single dumbbell appropriate for your fitness level and grip it in your left hand
- Kneel on the bench with your right knee. Plant your left on the floor
- Hinge at the hips to place your right hand on the bench.
- At this point, your back should be flat, head in a neutral position
- Rotate your left shoulder and bend your left elbow to place the length of your upper arm parallel to the floor
- There should be a right angle between the front of your upper left arm and lower left arm
- As you exhale, straighten your left arm whiles keeping your upper arm fixed in the start position to bring the dumbbell up and past the side of your lower body
- Once at the top of movement, inhale and return to the start position. This completes one rep
- Once you have completed a set, repeat on the opposite side

Extra info:

As with many dumbbell exercises, this one can be tricky to master. The key to getting this right is often awareness of the upper arm position. It's common for the upper arm to drop during the set. This will significantly reduce the training effect on the triceps. Before starting each rep, reassess your position.

Tricep extension with barbell

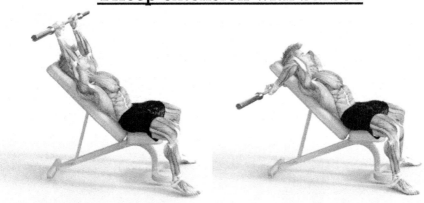

Description:

- You will need an incline workout bench or solid incline chair for this exercise
- Set up a barbell with an appropriate resistance for your fitness level and sit on the incline bench
- Grip the bar with an overhand grip so your hands are about shoulder width apart
- Raise the bar above your head with straight arms
- Keep your back flat to the bench and elbows facing forward
- As you inhale, bend at the elbows while keeping your upper arms fixed in the starting position and elbows facing forward
- The bar will lower behind your head and you should feel the stretch in your triceps. Once you reach full range of motion, exhale and return to the start position
- This completes one rep

Extra info:

This exercise requires strict form. Before using this in a workout, I would advise that you have a good "mind muscle connection" and that you know how your triceps feel when they are being challenged sufficiently. It's very common for trainers to overestimate the amount of resistance that is needed for this movement. Too much weight can make it very tempting to lose form and use other muscle groups to complete the rep.

It is also possible to perform this exercise from a lying position. This version is commonly known as "skull crushers". The difference is that you use a flat bench and start from a barbell chest press position with your straight arms angled slightly above your head.

Abs & core

Crunches

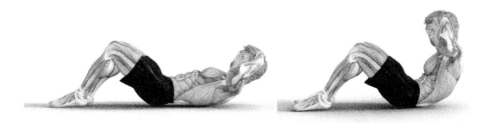

Description:

- Lie on your back on the floor or on a workout mat with your knees bent
- The soles of your feet should be flat on the floor
- Place your finger tips on the sides of your head
- Lift your shoulder blades up and away from the floor slightly by engaging your abdominals
- As you exhale, move your upper body towards your legs by hinging through your abdominal muscles
- Your lower back should remain in contact with the floor
- Once at the top of movement, inhale as your return to the start position

Extra info:

Bringing your feet closer to your glutes will make the exercise more challenging, but it will also help to ensure the movement has maximum focus on the abdominal muscles.

When returning to the start position between reps, it's important that your shoulder blades stay close, but do not make contact with the floor. This ensures that the engagement of the abdominal muscles stays active and gives more value to the set.

Crunches with resistance band

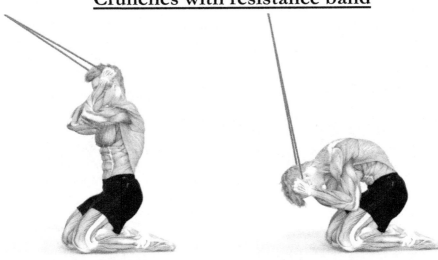

Description:

- Select a resistance band that's appropriate for your fitness level, loop through the door anchor and attach to the top of a door or other elevated anchor point
- Grip the ends of the band and place your fists by the side of your head
- Kneel on the floor, facing the door or anchor point
- Keep your back flat and head in a neutral position
- As you exhale, bring your elbows to your upper legs by bending your lower torso above your hips
- Once at maximum contraction, inhale as you return to the start position

Extra info:

This exercise is a bit trickier to get right for beginners when compared to crunches on the floor as more concentration is needed on the form.

Dorsal raises torso movement

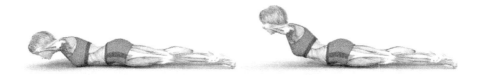

Description:

- Lie on the floor or an exercise mat face down and palace your fingers on your temples
- Lift your head and shoulders off the floor by engaging your back muscles
- The fronts of your feet should be in contact with the floor and your head should be in a neutral position
- As you exhale, slowly and under control, lift your upper body away from the floor by hyper extending through the lower back
- Once at the top of movement, hold for a second and return to the start position as you inhale

Extra info:

This is an exercise for the lower back. Lower back strength is important for everyone, especially if abdominals are strong. If you feel that your abs are strong, it is a good idea to add a lower back exercise to your workouts for balance. If you choose to use this exercise, I would advise adding it to the end of your workout or circuit training routine.

A strong, mobile lower back can help to prevent common back injuries, and this is a very accessible movement for most.

Advanced dorsal raises

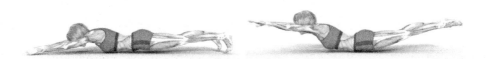

Description:

- Lie on the floor or an exercise mat face down. Also place your arms on the floor so they are straight in front of your head
- Lift your head, shoulders and outstretched arms off the floor by engaging your back muscles
- The fronts of your feet should be in contact with the floor and your head should be in a neutral position
- As you exhale, slowly and under control, lift your upper body and legs away from the floor by hyper extending through the lower back
- Your arms and legs should stay straight. Your pelvis and lower abdominals will remain in contact with the floor
- Once at the top of movement, hold for a second and return to the start position as you inhale

Extra info:

This is a more advanced version of the dorsal raise that provides the same benefits but gives more of a challenge by engaging more muscles of the posterior chain. If you are new to this type of movement, I would advise that you first become comfortable with the standard dorsal raise exercise.

Thank you! If you found this useful I'd like to help further…

First off, I would like to thank you for your purchase. It really means a lot that you spent your time on this guide. I am a self-published author with a passion for training and helping people get to where they want to be with fitness and by reading; you are supporting me and fuelling my passion.

This guide should give you a brilliant start in the world of bodyweight training and the planning that goes with it. But this is not my first fitness book! I've been writing and self-publishing for several years. I've written books on fitness motivation, planning, bodybuilding, home workouts and long distance running. These guides are based on my experience and formal education.

I've been a long distance endurance runner, a competing bodybuilder, and I have worked with personal training clients to change their lives through fitness, so I have a lot to share.

If you found this short guide useful and would like to read more about body transformations, fitness motivation, home workouts or more about resistance training and would like a clear path to follow, I have plenty more for you to look at including workbooks and journals for you to plan and track!

Most of my books are available in eBook and paperback format, and some are also available as audio titles narrated by an exceptional voice actor called Matt Addis.

Each fitness book is written as a standalone guide but also has its place as part of a series. So if you are a total beginner and want to become a bodybuilder or marathon runner as an end goal, I have you covered! Jump in at the start of the series with *"Fitness & Exercise Motivation"* and follow the steps, I'll be at the starting blocks with you and we will cross the finish line together!

If you would like to learn more about this series and my other books, you can do so by visiting my author page. Visit Amazon and search "James Atkinson", you will see my ugly mug, click it, and you should be taken to my page. Alternatively, just follow the link below - ☺

https://www.amazon.com/author/jamesatkinson

As we all know, diet plays a big part in health and fitness, and the two subjects fit hand in hand. So I would like to offer you a free download of seven healthy recipes that I created and use regularly myself. You can copy the recipes exactly, add your own twist to them, or simply take inspiration from them.

If you would like to grab this, you can do so by following the link below.

https://jimshealthandmuscle.com/healthy-recipes-sign-up

Remember The Podcast!

Trying to create an online business is tough, especially in the fitness niche! There is a lot of noise, "fairy-tale" fitness supplements, big personalities, and celebrities with huge online followings pushing their fitness ideas that often drown out the information that will actually make the difference.

In an attempt to widen my online reach, I created a podcast that is designed for the beginner who really wants to get results from their efforts. I set out to create bite sized podcast episodes of around twenty minutes that gave honest, actionable advice to the listener. This is still in its early stages, but I have to say that I've absolutely loved doing these podcast episodes and it is something that I plan to get stuck into more in the future.

If you are interested in fitness podcasts, you can find mine at

AudioFitTest.com

Or search Audiofittest wherever you get your podcasts from.

It would be great to have you along! If you do stop by, I would also really appreciate "Likes", "follows" and reviews. These things really help! The same goes for Amazon reviews for the books. If you have chance and you found the book useful, it would mean the world to me if you left a star rating and a short review.

Thanks again for your support and I wish you all the best with your training. Remember, I am always happy to help where I can, so if you have any questions, just give me a shout!

All the best,

Jim

Also by James Atkinson

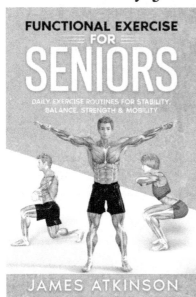

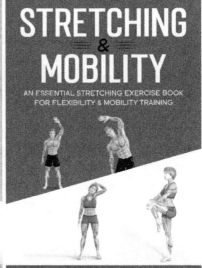

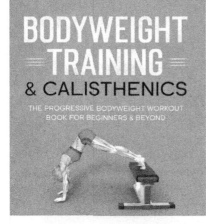

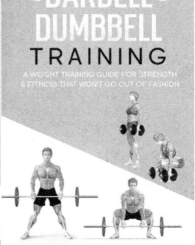

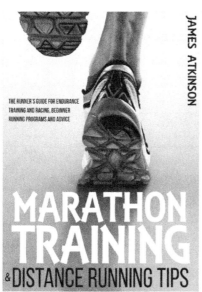

JAMES ATKINSON

THE RUNNER'S GUIDE FOR ENDURANCE TRAINING AND RACING, BEGINNER RUNNING PROGRAMS AND ADVICE

MARATHON TRAINING
&DISTANCE RUNNING TIPS

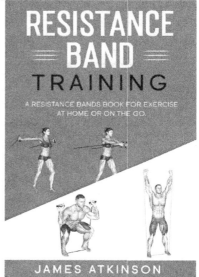

RESISTANCE BAND TRAINING

A RESISTANCE BANDS BOOK FOR EXERCISE AT HOME OR ON THE GO.

JAMES ATKINSON

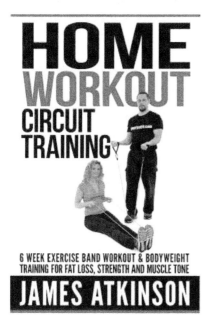

HOME WORKOUT
CIRCUIT TRAINING

6 WEEK EXERCISE BAND WORKOUT & BODYWEIGHT TRAINING FOR FAT LOSS, STRENGTH AND MUSCLE TONE

JAMES ATKINSON

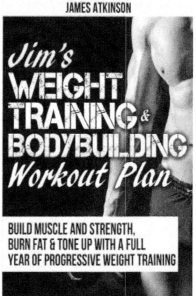

JAMES ATKINSON

Jim's **WEIGHT TRAINING & BODYBUILDING** *Workout Plan*

BUILD MUSCLE AND STRENGTH, BURN FAT & TONE UP WITH A FULL YEAR OF PROGRESSIVE WEIGHT TRAINING

Blank Program Cards

SETS & REPS			

ROUTINE #			

MUSCLE GROUP	EXERCISE	SETS	REPS

WEEKS	MON	TUE	WED	THURS	FRI	SAT	SUN
1							
2							
3							
4							
5							
6							

138

SETS & REPS			

ROUTINE #		

MUSCLE GROUP	EXERCISE	SETS	REPS

WEEKS	MON	TUE	WED	THURS	FRI	SAT	SUN
1							
2							
3							
4							
5							
6							

CIRCUIT TRAINING			

ROUTINE #			

MUSCLE GROUP	EXERCISE	REPS	SETS

WEEKS	MON	TUE	WED	THURS	FRI	SAT	SUN
1							
2							
3							
4							
5							
6							

CIRCUIT TRAINING			

ROUTINE #		

MUSCLE GROUP	EXERCISE	REPS	SETS

WEEKS	MON	TUE	WED	THURS	FRI	SAT	SUN
1							
2							
3							
4							
5							
6							

2 DAY SPLIT

ROUTINE #		

MUSCLE GROUP	EXERCISE	SETS	REPS
WORKOUT A			
WORKOUT B			

WEEKS	MON	TUE	WED	THURS	FRI	SAT	SUN
1							
2							
3							
4							
5							
6							

2 DAY SPLIT			

ROUTINE #			

MUSCLE GROUP	EXERCISE	SETS	REPS
WORKOUT A			
WORKOUT B			

WEEKS	MON	TUE	WED	THURS	FRI	SAT	SUN
1							
2							
3							
4							
5							
6							

143

Printed in Great Britain
by Amazon